Homemade Blended Formula Handbook

Marsha Dunn Klein M.Ed., OTR/L
Suzanne Evans Morris, Ph.D., CCC

Foreward by
Ellyn Satter, M.S., R.D.,CICSW, BCD

Published by
Mealtime Notions, LLC

Tucson, Arizona

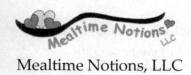

Mealtime Notions, LLC

Content and editorial by Marsha Dunn Klein and Suzanne Evans Morris.
Graphics and computer layout by Christine M. Streiff Sternberg
Editorial assistance by Christina Ravashiere Medvescek.

Printed in the United States of America by Mealtime Notions, LLC

Distributed by Mealtime Notions, LLC.
The Mealtime Notions website address is www.mealtimenotions.com
Ordering information is found on website.
Mealtime Notions, LLC, PO 35432, Tucson, AZ 85740.
Phone 520 829 9635 or fax 520 829 9636

Library of Congress Cataloging in Publication Data

ISBN 13: 978-0-692-65124-7

Homemade Blended Formula Handbook is a series of chapters on related topics which are woven together by common themes. After the book is read in its entirely, we expect readers will share specific reproducible sections with families and colleagues , so each individual topic is written to be able to be read as part of a whole as well as independent of the whole. Many chapters provide other resources that may help the reader who has further interest in that topic.

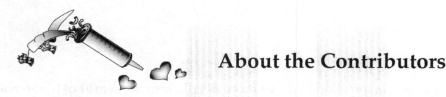

About the Contributors

Marsha Dunn Klein, ME d., OTR/L

Marsha is a pediatric occupational therapist from Tucson, AZ who specializes in feeding with infants and young children. She has coauthored *Feeding and Nutrition for the Child with Special Needs* with Tracy Delaney; *Pre-Feeding Skills, a Comprehensive Resource for Mealtime Development (1st and 2nd Editions)* and *Mealtime Participation Guide*, with Suzanne Evans Morris. She currently maintains a private practice in Tucson, Arizona at Mealtime Connections, LLC, www.mealtimeconnections.com and is the founder of Mealtime Notions, LLC. She has created feeding videos and DVD's entitled *Tube Feedings are Mealtimes Too, The Journey from Tube Feeding Towards Oral Feeding, Taking Tube Feedings to School,* and *The Get Permission Approach to Mealtimes and Oral Motor Treatment.* She is the designer and producer of the Duo♥Spoon™. She can be reached through her website, www.mealtimenotions.com.

Suzanne Evans Morris,P hD ,C CC

Suzanne is a speech-language pathologist in private practice near Charlottesville, VA. She is recognized nationally and internationally for her work in identifying and treating pre-speech and feeding disorders in young children. Suzanne is the director of New Visions, an organization that sponsors workshops for teaching feeding related skills and provides family related services and family oriented clinical services. She has written extensively about assessment and remediation techniques for children who have oral feeding problems. She has coauthored *Pre-Feeding Skills, a Comprehensive Resource for Mealtime Development (1st and 2nd Editions)* and *Mealtime Participation Guide*, with Marsha Dunn Klein. She can be reached through her website, www.new-vis.com.

Jude Trautlein, BA , B.S., R.D.

Jude is a registered dietitian with Your Nutrition Coach, LLC. She has over 15 years experience working with children and their families, particularly children with special health care needs and g-tubes.

Ellen Duperret, B.S., R.D.

Ellen has been a Registered Dietitian since 1982. She has specialized in nutrition for children with developmental disabilities since 1995. She, along with Marsha Dunn Klein and Jude Trautlein, is the co-author of several articles on homemade blended formulas for children with tubes through *Nutrition Focus* and *Exceptional Parent Magazine.*

Sanford Newmark, MD .

Dr. Newmark is a physician with over 20 years of experience in pediatrics. He has completed a 2-year fellowship in Integrative Medicine at the Program in Integrative Medicine at the University of Arizona under the leadership of Dr. Andrew Weil. He maintains a consulting practice in Pediatric Integrative Medicine in Tucson, Arizona. He can be reached through the Center for Pediatric Integrative Medicine in Tucson, Arizona and at his website www.doctornewmark.com.

Parent Contributors

Lisa Larsen

Lisa is Bella's mother. She was our inspiration to delve more deeply into the world of homemade blended formulas and share information with others. Because Bella experienced gastrointestinal discomfort and allergies, Lisa created a homemade blended formula for her daughter at a time when her physicians and dietitians had little experience with it. With the initial encouragement and guidance of a therapist, she painstakingly added foods to Bella's diet, until the diet was all foods. She has generously shared her experiences with countless other families. Thank you! Bella, now 13 is a fully oral and enthusiastic eater!

Fran McDermott

Fran is Thomas' mother. Thomas has had a feeding tube since infancy due to gastrointestinal and swallowing difficulties. He also has multiple food allergies. With the help of her dietitian, Fran has created a blended formula from commercial baby foods that works well for Thomas. At ten, he is both comfortable and enthusiastic about taking small tastes of food by mouth and participating in family and school mealtimes.

Jenn Sandman

Jenn is Harper's mother. Harper received a gastrostomy tube because of complications from gastroesophageal reflux and stomach pain. He has been receiving a homemade blended formula with a carefully planned vegetarian diet. He, at three and a half, is well on his way to eating all foods orally.

Tina Valente

Tina is Joey's mother. Joey received a nasogastric tube at eight months of age and a gastrostomy tube shortly after that because of complications from a rare liver disease. At nine, Joey still has his tube and he and his mother still enjoy creating a rich tube diet of homemade blended foods.

Trish Whitehouse

Trish is Bobby's mother. Bobby received a nasogastric tube and then a gastrostomy tube due to complications from cardiac conditions and surgery. She had positive experiences involving the whole family in the process of creating homemade blended formulas. Bobby, now six, is off his tube, and is a fully oral eater.

About Our Foreword Contributor

Ellyn Satter, M.S., R.D., CICSW, BCD is an internationally recognized authority on eating and feeding. Her books, journal and magazine articles, teaching materials, seminars and media interviews have made her well-known to the lay public, professionals and the media as the leading authority on nutrition and feeding of infants and children. The author of the division of responsibility in feeding (parents are responsible for the *what, where and when of feeding,* children are responsible for the *how much and whether of eating),* Satter has led nutrition, health and mental health professionals as well as the general public to adopt wise and emotionally healthy approaches to feeding and eating. She can be reached through her website www.ellynsatter.com .

About Our Editor

Christina Ravashiere Medvescek is the Director of Editorial Services for the Muscular Dystrophy Association of the United States and mother of three children including one with multiple disabilities.

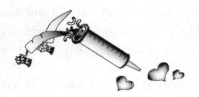

Foreword
Ellyn Satter, M.S., R.D., CICSW, BCD

Feeding is about relationship. Feeding is more than picking out food and getting it into a child. Eating is more than throwing wood on a fire or pumping gas into a car. Eating and feeding reflect our attitudes and relationships with ourselves and with others as well as our histories. Eating is about our regard for ourselves, our connection with our bodies and our commitment to life itself. Feeding your child is about the love and connection between you and your child, about trusting or controlling, about providing or neglecting, about accepting or rejecting. Eating can be joyful, full of zest and vitality. Or it can be fearful, bounded by control and avoidance. The *Homemade Blended Formula Handbook* will help you make feeding your child joyful and rewarding.

The bottom line is family meals. Children and adolescents who have regular family meals do better in all ways—nutritionally, academically, socially and emotionally, with respect to avoidance of overweight, eating disorders, and avoidance of early drug usage and sexual behavior. Family meals have more to do with positive outcomes for children and adolescents than any other factor—extra-curricular activities, church, tutors, music lessons—you name it.

The *Homemade Blended Formula Handbook* shows you how to include your tube-fed child in family meals. Klein and Morris are tuned in to children and parents. Throughout their careers, they have sought ways to make feeding as positive and rewarding as can be. In the *Homemade Blended Formula Handbook* they share methods and insights, and they share stories. The stories tell us about what it means to a child to be included—to *not* be different. We take for granted sharing food and eating together. Children who *can't* participate show us just how important it is. Children are delighted when they are included in family mealtimes by being offered family foods—whether they simply touch and smell the food, lick and taste, or ingest blended family food through a tube.

Feeding children demands a division of responsibility. As I illustrated in *Child of Mine, Feeding with Love and Good Sense*, feeding is *good* parenting when parents do the *what, when* and *where* of feeding and allow their child to do the *how much* and *whether* of eating. Sharing responsibility during feeding with a tube fed child maintains a sense of connected give-and-take during feeding. Too often, that connection is spoiled when parents are told the exact amount of tube feeding formula a child shall consume. The irony is that those precise instructions are based on educated guesses—rough calculations. We simply can't predict how many calories a given child will need. Calorie needs vary widely from one child to the next and from one day to the next. The only way you can accurately know how much a child *should* eat is by observing how much the child *does* eat. A child who needs few calories will be full and satisfied on those few calories, even if he takes in less than the instructions say. The child who needs a lot of calories will only be satisfied on those many calories, even if she takes in more than the instructions say.

I watched in horror during a clinical assessment as parents pumped the "required" amount of formula into their 17-month-old daughter. At first, the child sat in her high chair and played happily enough. Then she started to squirm. Then her face turned red and she began to retch. "See her reflux?" said her concerned mother. The tube feeding inexorably continued although the child slumped in her chair, looking dazed. At long last the prescribed amount of formula was gone. When she was taken out of the high chair, the miserable and half-stunned child staggered to her father's lap, where she slumped for a full half hour before she recovered enough to resume playing. Have you ever felt so stuffed with food that you were absolutely miserable? That is how that child felt after every tube feeding.

We worry that our children won't get enough to eat, and we worry most about our medically vulnerable children. For health professionals as well as parents, it is a great risk to trust the child to determine *how much* and to guide feeding based on information coming from the child. In the *Homemade Blended Formula Handbook*, Klein and Morris thinkingly and wisely take that risk. They remind you that children who are fed by tube are as capable as any other child of doing their part with determining *how much* they need to eat and can therefore show us when they are hungry and when are full. Our job is to guide feeding based on their indicators of hunger and fullness.

Tube fed children have subtle and often-unusual indicators of hunger and fullness. My 17-month-old was full somewhere before she started to squirm. When her parents looked at her cues, they discovered that she was hungry when she became cranky and whiny and wouldn't look at them, and she was full when she relaxed, stopped playing and began begging to get down from her high chair. My small patient learned to eat by mouth a few weeks after that assessment, so I can't tell you the impact on tube feeding of their more tuned-in approach. I do know her "reflux" went away—it had been the product of overstuffing.

The part where you balance your *what* with the child's *whether* is trickier, and you must become nutritionally sophisticated to do your part with feeding. You have to understand nutrition and food composition to provide your child with a formula that has an appropriate number of calories per ounce and satisfies your child's requirements for protein, vitamins, minerals, trace elements, fatty acids and water. Klein and Morris have you covered on this, as well. As the parents in this book illustrate, once they learn the rules for putting together blended formulas, they cautiously begin to improvise by increasing the variety of components in tube feeding recipes and by blending family meals into a consistency that the child can manage.

Which brings us to the consideration of mealtimes for the rest of the family. If the tube fed child is to join the family table via homemade blended formulas, there must be a family table for that child to join. If the child is to join the family, period, that child must to the greatest extent possible be treated the same as the other children in the family—no more or less special than anyone else. Both require the structure of regular family meals. To keep up the considerable day-in-day-out effort of providing family meals, build meals around foods that you find richly rewarding to plan, prepare and eat. Then make meals enjoyable by letting your family members pick and choose from what is available, eating as much or as little as they want, even if they want to eat only 2 or 3 foods. I wrote about "Orchestrating Family Meals" in *Secrets of Feeding a Healthy Family*. With a little help from an experienced dietitian, parents who have developed a good sense of variety, balance and proportion have gotten to the point where they matter-of-factly prepare homemade blended formulas for their tube fed child on a meal-by-meal basis. You can too.

Most important of all, relax and enjoy your child. After all, why would any of us have children if we didn't expect to have fun?

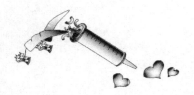

Acknowledgements

Children and families will always be our teachers. There are so many children who have tubes and families who have lovingly learned to use them. They have been the pioneers in discussions of homemade blended formulas. So many of these families have shared their personal stories, experiences and techniques with us so we, in turn, could share them with you, our reader.

A special group of mothers who participated in the Feeding and G-tube listservs volunteered to complete two detailed questionnaires. Their thoughtful answers and shared experiences provided the major guidelines for the format and content of this book. We offer our deepest appreciation for the contributions of Jane Barker, Kim Brownen, Caroline Daley, Rose-Marie Gallagher, Jennifer Hisrich, Pam Lahr, Leslie Diane Marino, Tawnia Richie, Rachel Trindle, and Sharon Williamson.

We would like to especially acknowledge the very personal and important contributions made by Jenn Sandman, mother of Harper, Lisa Larson, mother of Bella, Fran McDermott, mother of Thomas, Tina Valente, mother of Joey, and Trish Whitehouse, mother of Bobby. Each of these mothers found a way to make peace with the feeding tube and provide incredible nutrition with homemade blended formulas. Each found her own way to provide the homemade meals and then generously give of her time to write down her experiences to share with other families.

This book could not have been written without the contributions and hours of content support and review provided by Ellen Duperret, R.D., and Jude Trautlein, R.D. They have been willing to learn with families and other professionals as we have gained experience and understanding about homemade blended formulas. Their strong nutrition foundation has increased our overall understanding of how to provide homemade blended formulas and why they work for so many families.

Special thanks also to Sanford Newark, M.D. He has helped us understand the medical aspects of homemade blended formulas and helped other doctors learn about it and give it a chance.

Thanks to Chris Sternberg who patiently took our ideas and our drafts and turned them into a book with a cover! We appreciate the hours of painstaking work. We appreciated the editorial comments from a number of colleagues and would like to especially thank Kim Edwards, OTR/L, Mandy Guendelsberg, OTR/L, Robyn Lundeen COTA/L, Cuyler Romeo, OTR/L, Janet Toney, OTR/L.

Special thanks to Jenn Ferguson and Amanda Whitney for revision and CD support.

Marsha and Suzanne

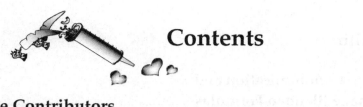

Contents

II. Tube Feeding Mealtimes

III. Nutritional Needs

IV. Preparing Homemade Blended Formulas

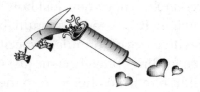

Introduction

Many families who are providing tube feedings for their children have asked, "Why can't I feed this child the nutrition I feed my other children?" or "What can I offer my child besides the same formula every day?" or "How would I go about providing real blended food through the tube?" or "Can I still use the commercial formula and just add a little food?" or "Where would I start"?

These families have often asked dietitians, pediatricians and other feeding team members these questions, only to have them admit to having little or no experience with blended foods in tube feedings. Much to the frustration of families, many of these professionals have asked them, "Why would you want to offer something besides commercial formula?" Some professionals have said, "Well, I've never had anyone ask that question, but let's learn together." This handbook is for them, all of them: families who ask "why?" "how?" and "what?" and the professionals who have limited experiences and want to learn. It provides a starting point for making homemade blended formulas and a sharing of information, based on what we already know about feeding children. It incorporates what we know about mealtime experiences and what helps children grow. It combines this knowledge with the experiences of parents and other professionals who have written these chapters.

What is a Homemade Blended Formula?

Historically, these types of tube feeding formulas have been called "blender feedings," "blenderized formula," or "blenderized tube feedings." We have added the word "homemade" to celebrate the personal and nurturing nature of the preparation. We define a homemade blended formula as any formula that a parent makes that modifies a standard formula with "real "foods. It could be a commercial formula with a small amount of baby food fruit or vegetable added, or three meals a day of blended food with commercial formula at night, or a complete diet of homemade blended foods, or many options in between. We would have preferred to title the book "Homemade Blended Meals" to remind readers that tube feedings are mealtimes too. However, "Homemade Blended Formula" clarifies that the book is directed towards the needs of parents and professionals who share the lives of tube fed children.

Historical Perspective

Tube feedings have been around in some form for a long time. The use of gastrostomy tubes, knowledge of the digestive system and nutrition, and the technology of tube feedings has developed over centuries. In the 60s and early 70s, when many of us began supporting families of tube fed children, there were far fewer tubes, so our experience with tube feedings was limited. Only the sickest children received supplemental feedings. Tubes were predominantly limited to larger catheter tubes. Infants received tube feedings with their infant formulas. However, as they grew, their parents added baby foods to the formula or pureed family foods and did the best they could to get the food through the tube. Our collective experience was predominantly "blenderized feedings."

By the mid 1970s, formula companies developed specialized tube formulas based on detailed nutritional research, which provided a better understanding of micronutrients and total nutritional daily requirements. Families moved from blending table foods to the use of commercial formulas. These formulas became an easier option for families. Dietitians and physicians supported the use of these formulas because they offered nutrition based on the newest research. They knew just how many calories, macronutrients and micronutrients the child was receiving. It was easily quantifiable, very portable, pasteurized and balanced. Families were sent home with cases of formula, a specific time schedule, and a prescribed number of ounces per feeding. Tube feedings often became just one more procedure required of parents when their medically fragile children returned home from the hospital. The tube feeding process and its vocabulary of doses and ounces and mls or ccs inadvertently emphasized the medical nature of nutrition and increased the separation from the family meal and the feeding relationship that parents dreamt of for their children.

Today, technology has greatly changed and made tube feedings much easier for children and their families. They're more portable, more efficient and less restrictive. We also have become a more health-conscious and better-informed society. We're learning daily from research literature and the popular press about foods we should add or remove from our diets. We're increasing our understanding of the importance of diversified diets as the best way to provide the micronutrients needed for optimum health. Parents are rightfully asking if one formula, one diet or one recipe can provide all the nutritional variation needed to maximize nutrition, health and growth for their tube fed children.

In addition many parents are asking about homemade blended formulas as a way to empower themselves in making personal choices about foods. Many parents report that preparing homemade blended formulas gives them more control in their children's growth and feeding, and allows them to nurture their tube fed children with food as they would orally fed children.

In this handbook, we consider how to integrate the best of past technologies and concepts with the present, to create a new present and future for tube fed children and their families. We'd like to help families and professionals think about the meaning of tube feedings and find ways to integrate them into the family mealtime.

Research

Very few published articles describe the "hows" and "whys" of homemade blended formulas. By contrast, a great deal has been researched about healthy nutrition for orally fed children.

We have a large amount of information about what to feed children, how much to feed them at different ages, what nutrients are needed for optimal growth and how to interact with children at mealtimes. There's limited research on how to translate this information for tube fed children and their nutrition, and it's dominated by information about commercial formulas and their benefits.

Commercial formulas need not be the only option. Many parents are feeding their children homemade blended formulas and have had very positive experiences. Instead of being written up in scientific journals, these positive experiences have been shared anecdotally through professional discussions and from parent to parent by phone, Internet mailing lists and online chat rooms. We need to encourage and support research about homemade blended formulas. Historically, good research is designed from a broad collection of personal and clinical experiences, which enables researchers to ask meaningful questions.

We've seen the changes that homemade blended formulas have made for many children and their families. In this handbook, we've included input from families in the United States, Canada, England and Australia, obtained from professional clinical experiences, informal parent questionnaires and feeding support groups on the Internet. It's hoped that the experiences and questions raised in this handbook will inspire researchers to ask those meaningful questions.

Team Approach

It's our belief and experience that supporting families in the decision-making process necessary for making homemade blended formulas requires a team approach. The parent is the leader of the team. We trust the instincts and knowledge of parents as they make everyday decisions about feeding their orally fed children. And we need to trust parents of tube fed children to make nutritional decisions for their children.

The special considerations of tube feeding technology and special diets, and the translation of oral feeding knowledge to tube feeding, often requires additional team support. When parents are considering serving homemade blended formulas, it's very important to work closely with their children's health care team, starting with the primary care physician.

To reflect that team support in this guide, in addition to our own years of clinical experiences as an occupational therapist and speech-language pathologist, we've compiled and edited articles from dietitians, physicians, and most importantly, parents. Parents have written articles and given input every step along the way. They've suggested topics, provided information, reviewed drafts and given feedback.

It's our intent to provide information about feeding children, education about homemade blended formulas, guidelines for introducing blended foods through the tube and guidelines for creating your own formula. We'll share parent and professional experiences. But mealtimes are personal in nature, whether they're oral or tube mealtimes. What works for one family and one child may not work well for another family and child. We include guidelines for providing blended meals through a tube, but more importantly we share ways to listen to your child and move forward in offering food as your child indicates readiness. Each child and family is different.

The choices families make in their journeys with tube feeding reflect their family circumstances and dynamics, and their children's specific nutritional needs. No equipment or diet defines what makes mealtimes work. The essence of the tube feeding mealtime lies in the bigger picture. Positive and successful mealtimes are defined by how tube feedings are offered, how blended foods are introduced, how cues are read, and how we listen to children.

It's not our perspective that every child who receives tube feedings should be given a homemade blended formula. Rather, it's our intent to offer information so parents and professionals can make informed choices for feeding children who receive nutrition through a feeding tube.

Marsha Dunn Klein
Suzanne Evans Morris

3

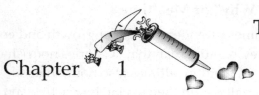

Tube Feedings are Mealtimes, Too!

Chapter 1

Marsha Dunn Klein, M.Ed., OTR/L

Making the decision to have a feeding tube placed in a child for supplemental feeding can be an emotional one. Parents describe ranges of reactions that go from relief to sadness, and from grief to confusion.

A caring hospital or clinic staff will review all the technical aspects of tube feedings with families before sending them home to do it on their own. They will describe how to use the equipment, the routine, the timing, the formula, the ounces or mls/ccs, the syringes and the pumps.

There's a great deal to learn and remember, and it's easy for families to become overwhelmed and return home scared and worried. It's easy to completely focus on the technical "procedural" aspects of tube feeding because parents want to do it right! Many parents stop thinking of the tube feeding as a meal at all, and present the formula as one more medical procedure to be fit into the day. The "procedure" becomes central and the "mealtime" becomes lost.

But these tube feedings <u>are</u> the child's mealtimes. Let's look at many of the ways parents can turn tube feedings into the type of mealtime they might experience with any child.

What is a Mealtime?

Mealtimes are times to take in calories, but they are much more than that. The meaning of, and feelings about, "mealtimes" can vary from situation to situation depending on where we eat, with whom we eat, why we eat, when we eat, and what we eat. A mealtime at a family dinner table may feel different from a fast-food breakfast in the car on the way to school. Meals take on different meanings when food is offered at a business meeting, picnic, romantic anniversary, birthday celebration, or family reunion. As the participants

and purposes of mealtimes change, so does the atmosphere of the mealtime.

Let's look at the "where," "who," "why," "when" and "what "of mealtimes and see if there are ways to share all of these aspects of oral mealtimes with tube fed children.

The "Where" of Mealtime

For orally fed children, the "where" of mealtimes evolves from parents' arms to the highchair to the family table, as children gain skills in eating. The "where " of tube fed meals evolves in the same manner, from being held or fed in an infant seat to sitting at the family table.

Feeding orally fed babies is a time of closeness, a cuddle time, a time of togetherness. Often parents and babies look into each other's eyes and fall in love during feedings. Even though tube feedings are given by pump or syringe, this physical and emotional closeness still can be created. Babies can be held intimately in a parent's arms in the same general positions used for offering the breast or bottle. Some mothers hold the baby close to the breast for some calming skin-to-skin time during the tube feeding. Others feed their baby in an infant seat so hands are free for tube feeding paraphernalia. This still allows for that face-to-face togetherness.

Parents come up with many creative ways to achieve physical closeness while still holding formulas and syringes. Velcro® fasteners, shoelaces, safety pins and tape have all been used to provide the parent with the "extra hand" needed for comfort and success.

For older children, mealtimes take place in a high chair or booster seat or at the family table. Receiving tube feedings during meals shared with family members gives children the opportunity to associate tummy fullness with the smells, sights, sounds and textures of mealtime. It gives them the opportunity to learn from watching others interact with food, so that some of their mealtime exploration is inspired by imitation.

Many families offer oral foods just before or during the tube meal at the family table. Some families use a feeding pump and others use a syringe to put food in the tube. Both of these can be kept out of sight, so children can begin to view themselves as oral feeders as they explore tastes.

The "where" of mealtimes can be in places other than the family table. Parents find ways to take tube meals with them to picnics, friends' houses or the mall. They discover ways to travel and efficiently offer tube meals at hotels or restaurants. With time and experience, most families find ways to vary the "where" of mealtimes so the child fed by tube experiences mealtimes in many places.

The "Who" of Mealtime

Orally fed children eat with many different people: mothers, fathers, brothers and sisters, grandparents, aunts and uncles, cousins and friends. Tube fed children can receive their nourishment with different people too. But all too often, one parent ends up being the only person who can do the tube feedings. No one else develops the skills or confidence. This can create a great deal of pressure on the parent and the child.

From the beginning, it's helpful for all of the child's caregivers to learn and practice providing tube meals. With practice, different people can share in the feeding responsibilities and mealtime interactions.

Children learn from eating with others. They learn to imitate the mechanics of eating as well as the conversations and social interactions of mealtimes. Siblings provide wonderful role models. When tube feeding mealtimes are shared with several other people, there's a greater social atmosphere and the tube fed child often feels more included and relaxed.

The "Why" of Mealtime

Mealtimes provide calories for growth and energy, but they're more than that. Calories nourish us physically, but mealtimes also nourish us emotionally, with their social, interactive and communicative opportunities.

When we share meals with others we have opportunities for rich interaction and communication. Families may discuss what happened at school or work, the pending visit of a grandparent, current events or family plans for the weekend. Children have opportunities to learn social rules such as manners, turn taking, consideration for others, mealtime preparation and routines. The content may vary, but the interaction and shared communication is there.

Tube fed children receive needed calories for growth from tube feedings, but they also can be richly nourished by their mealtime interactions with others.

The "When" of Mealtime

The "when" of mealtimes evolves from infancy through childhood. Infants typically are fed according to a routine that's a blend of demand and scheduled mealtimes. Initially, they may be fed when they express hunger through crying. Parents modify this pattern by gradually stretching out feeding times to create a more predictable and reasonable schedule. Alternatively, babies initially may be fed every three or four hours on an inflexible schedule that gradually becomes more variable as they're able to give a wider range of hunger cues and parents learn to read those cues. As infants mature into toddlers, their mealtime schedule gradually blends into the family mealtime schedule.

Parents ultimately decide the "when" of mealtimes, but their decisions are guided by feedback from the child. Some orally fed children give feedback that they need to eat only three large meals a day; others need five or six smaller meals or a schedule of three good-sized main meals and two or three small between-meal snacks. Parents learn this by watching and offering food and ultimately deciding upon a mealtime routine that optimizes the child's comfort, attitude, appetite and growth.

It works the same for tube feedings. Parents listen and adjust. Some children need bolus meals by day and more extended drip feedings at night to be comfortable. Others need daytime feedings every four hours because a three-hour schedule places stress on their gastrointestinal system. Others become cranky unless they're fed every three hours. Some children can easily be fed at the same time the family eats, while others need to work into that option more slowly because they're overwhelmed by the group mealtime situation.

The "What" of Mealtime

Adults are in charge of the menu at mealtimes. It's their responsibility to prepare foods that meet their child's nutritional and developmental needs. Orally fed children are in charge of how much they eat. As they learn to enjoy solid foods and have more food choices, they then are in charge of how much they'll eat and which foods served at the meal they'll eat.

For many families, the "what" provided in the tube is a commercial formula. Most tube fed children don't have a choice of "what" or "how much." Many parents also have felt they haven't had these choices as they've followed the strict recommendations of their medical teams. When families want to change the "what" of tube feedings, they begin to ask questions about homemade blended formulas.

Many parents describe feeling more comfortable and connected with their children when they have more choices and can make many of their own decisions about their child's nutrition. They become partners in mealtime decisions rather than technicians offering a "dose" of food. Parents describe the relief of being able to walk down the baby food aisle in the grocery store and pick favorite foods for their child. They describe positive feelings as they offer this type of dietary diversity.

Working with the health care team to add some type of blended food to their child's tube feeding routine can empower parents as they begin to make some decisions in the "what" of their child's tube meals.

For additional information on tube feeding mealtime concepts see:

Klein, M.D. (2003). *Tube Feedings are Mealtimes, Too!* VHS & DVD.
Tucson, AZ: Mealtime Notions, LLC (www.mealtimenotions.com).

Klein, M.D. (2007). Turn Those Tube Feedings into Mealtimes!
Exceptional Parent Magazine, 36:06 (February).

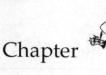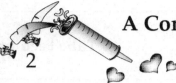

A Comparison of Oral and Tube Feeding Meals

Chapter 2

Marsha Dunn Klein, M.Ed., OTR/L
Suzanne Evans Morris, Ph.D, CCC

To increase the comfort level of tube feeding meals, let's explore the multiple ways tube feedings are similar to oral feedings, and what we know works when feeding children.

Component of Feeding	Oral Feeding	Tube Feeding
Closeness	Babies who eat by mouth are held in parents' arms for feeding so they can look into each other's eyes.	Tube fed babies can be fed in parents' arms or face-to-face in an infant seat, so parent and child can look into each other's eyes.
Positioning	Babies and children who eat by mouth are held in their parents' arms for feeding and moved to the highchair and finally the table.	Tube fed babies can be held in their parent's arms, or face-to-face in an infant seat for feeding, and moved to the highchair and finally the table.
Mealtime Partners	Children who eat by mouth can have multiple feeders and mealtime partners. These may include the child's mother, father, siblings, grandparents, relatives and friends.	Tube fed children can have multiple feeders and mealtime partners. These may include the child's mother, father, siblings, grandparents, relatives and friends.
Trust	Children who eat by mouth learn to trust their mealtime partners when these adults show them respect. They learn that when they're hungry they'll be fed, and when they're full they'll be allowed to stop. They trust that they can count on their grown ups.	Tube fed children learn to trust the adults who feed them when their mealtime partners show them respect. They need to know that they can feel comfortable during meals and that they'll be fed enough to grow and thrive. They also need to know that they won't be fed too much and will be listened to when they've had enough.
Communication	Children who eat by mouth communicate their mealtime hunger, thirst, fullness, pace and preferences with body movements, facial and eye expressions, sounds and words. Mealtimes work best if adults listen.	Tube fed children communicate their mealtime hunger, thirst, fullness, pace and preferences with body movements, facial and eye expressions, sounds and words. Mealtimes work best if adults listen.
Socialization	Children who eat by mouth learn to enjoy the company of other people and expand their encounters with food into the community. They go to the grocery store, restaurants, schools, picnics and parties.	Tube fed children learn to enjoy the company of other people and expand their encounters with food into the community. They go to the grocery store, restaurants, schools, picnics and parties.

Component of Feeding	Oral Feeding	Tube Feeding
Imitation	Children who eat by mouth learn a great deal about mealtimes from watching others eat and enjoy eating.	Tube fed children learn a great deal about mealtimes from watching others eat and enjoy eating.
Adult & Child Roles	It's the adult's job to provide the "what, where and when" of mealtimes. It's the child's job to decide "how much," "which foods" and "whether to eat".	It's the adult's job to provide the "what, where and when" of tube mealtimes. It's the child's job to let them know "how much" and guide the pace of the meal to support maximal comfort.
Appetite	Children who eat by mouth eat when they're hungry and stop when they're full. Their food intake varies from meal to meal and day to day as they grow.	When we read the cues of tube fed children, we can offer formula until they're full and vary the amount of formula from meal to meal and day to day as they grow.
Food Familiarization	Children who eat by mouth often need to be around new food tastes and textures multiple times before they feel familiar enough to eat them.	Tube fed children often need to be around new food tastes and textures multiple times before they feel familiar enough to taste and eat them.
Pace	Children who eat by mouth pace themselves during the meal, pausing when necessary for comfort and socialization. They never eat a meal with every bite taken at the same pace or rate of time.	Tube fed children need pacing during the meal for comfort and socialization. They can guide the speed and pacing of the meal by giving the person feeding them a cue to stop or start the flow of the formula.
Food Introduction	Children who eat by mouth transition from breast milk or formula to one new food at a time. If the new food agrees with them and they enjoy it, more foods are added one at a time. This slow introduction of food continues until the parent is confident that the child can enjoy and grow from a varied table food diet.	Tube fed children transition from breast milk or formula to a homemade blended formula one new food at a time. If the new food agrees with them, more foods are added one at a time until the parent is confident the child can enjoy and grow from a varied blended food diet.
Dietary Diversity	Babies who eat by mouth encounter a wide variety of tastes in breast milk. As their diet is expanded by the introduction of new foods, they receive the nutritional support they need. Children depend upon dietary diversity to obtain all of the nutrients needed for health and growth.	Tube fed babies initially receive breast milk or formula. They can receive a widely diverse diet from homemade blended foods offered through the tube. Blended foods can be tasted orally if the child can swallow safely, or tasted through burps.

Component of Feeding	Oral Feeding	Tube Feeding
Place Diversity	Children who eat by mouth eat in a variety of different settings (home, at the park, at homes of relatives and friends, in the car, at restaurants).	Tube fed children can receive their meals in a variety of different settings (home, at the park, at homes of relatives and friends, in the car, at restaurants).
Preferences	Children who eat by mouth have preferences. They let us know what they like and don't like.	Tube fed children have preferences. They let us know what they like and don't like as they move towards more food interactions.
Routine	Children who eat by mouth are fed in a daily routine that tends towards three meals and two or three snacks. Timing of individual meals may vary from day to day with family activities.	Tube fed children can be fed in a daily routine that mimics that of children who are fed by mouth. The timing of individual meals may vary with family activities.
Sensory Exploration	Children who eat by mouth constantly explore the sensory environment of food and utensils. They smell, poke, taste, touch, squish, smash and drop food.	Tube fed children need to learn about and become familiar and trusting of food by smelling, poking, tasting, touching, squishing, smashing and dropping food.
Skill Mastery	Children who eat by mouth are given the opportunity to explore and master the skills of eating new foods and using new utensils as they show readiness, interest, confidence and enjoyment.	Tube fed children need to be given the opportunity to explore and master the skills of eating new foods and using new utensils as they show readiness, interest, confidence and enjoyment.
Individual Nature	Each child is an individual and will let adults know their sensory preferences for new food tastes and textures. They show their readiness for spoons, forks, cups and straws. Adults help them move to the next steps in mealtime development as the child shows enjoyment, confidence and motivation.	Each child is an individual and will let adults know their sensory preferences for new food tastes and textures. They show their readiness for spoons, forks, cups and straws. Adults help them move to the next steps in mealtime development as the child shows enjoyment, confidence and motivation.

For additional information on mealtime characteristics and influences see:

Morris, S.E. and Klein, M.D. (2000). Chapters 1, 2 and 3. *Pre-feeding Skills – A Comprehensive Resource for Mealtime Development, 2nd ed.* Austin, TX: Pro-Ed.

Satter, Ellyn. (2000). *Child of Mine, Feeding with Love and Good Sense.* Boulder, CO. Bull Publishing Company.

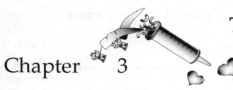

Chapter 3

The Continuum Concept in Homemade Blended Formulas

Marsha Dunn Klein, M.Ed., OTR/L

We use the term "homemade blended formula" to mean any formula that has been modified in a personal way with real foods to provide nutrition for a tube fed child.

The term suggests a continuum of meanings. We would call it a homemade blended formula if the family:

- added a pureed fruit to a commercial formula to increase fiber and assist in bowel formation and elimination;

- used a combination of commercial baby foods to offer three bolus meals during the day;

- provided a diet consisting of no commercial formula and only a blended combination of fruits, vegetables, protein, grains, dairy and oils;

- offered the child the family meal orally and then blended the remainder of the meal and provided it through the tube.

All of these options are homemade in that the parent modified the commercial formula with additions. All could be described as a homemade blended formula, and may be further described as a partial-food or total-food blended formula. In a sense, the term "homemade blended formula" suggests this continuum and the process of moving in the direction of total blended food meals.

Homemade Blended Formula Continuum

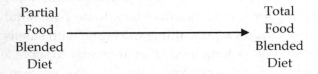

A homemade blended formula is food, real food. It is offered as a meal that happens to be given by tube instead of by mouth. We know a great deal about foods and we know about meals. We know

about what and how and when to feed children. If we focus on what we know about helping orally fed babies move from the breast and bottle toward table foods, we realize we already know a great deal about the homemade blended formula transition process.

Parents who want to experiment with homemade blended formulas should work closely with the child's medical team. By considering tube feedings as baby food and baby mealtimes and not as a medical procedure, parents, dietitians and pediatricians discover they know more about this process than they previously thought! They may feel less overwhelmed and much more confident as they contemplate the possibility of a homemade blended transition for their child.

Oral and Tube Meal Continuum

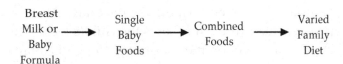

The generally accepted wisdom about helping infants transition from breast or bottle towards solids is that it's a gradual process. It often takes two to three years for families to feel that their children are orally eating a wide variety of food flavors and textures. It's not a quick transition where one day babies are getting all their calories from breast milk and the next day they're weaned and eating all table foods. It's a *process*.

Pediatricians generally recommend supplementing breast or bottle feeding with pureed baby food at six months, while still providing breast milk or formula for most of the calories. They suggest that parents offer one new baby food at a time, watch for allergies, observe the baby's reaction, and if the baby enjoys the process and seems to want more, then continue.

First foods are offered every three to five days to allow time to watch for allergic reactions. Gradually more new single-ingredient foods are added. Mixed dinners and combinations of different foods follow single foods. The variety of food flavors and texture challenges increases as breast milk and formula calories decrease. Eventually, as children show efficient and confident skills in eating, table foods are provided at family meals.

The transition of an orally fed baby from a liquid diet to solids can be seen as a continuum, with breast milk or baby formula at one end and a varied family diet including many flavors, textures and types of foods at the other end. In between are many combinations.

The introduction of a homemade blended formula also can be viewed as a *process*, a parallel continuum. Just as we make slow transitions for orally fed babies, we implement changes in a gradual way for tube fed children moving onto a homemade blended formula. Children are not on a commercial formula one day and then offered a completed blended formula the next day. The process takes time. It follows the child's lead. The child's final diet on the continuum depends totally on the child's response and the family's needs.

Food Choice Continuum

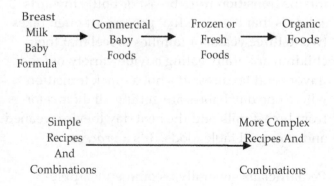

There are many food decisions to be made when orally fed babies move along the food continuum. These choices are personal, based on the individual needs and preferences of each child and family.

Preparation Continuum

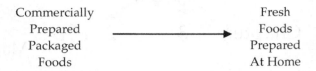

Some mothers choose breast milk, while others choose commercial baby formula. Others use a combination. As the baby indicates readiness for a pureed solid consistency, some families choose commercial baby food preparations while others offer homemade blended baby food. Parents who choose to make their own baby foods may blend frozen or fresh fruits and vegetables while others provide only fresh organic fruits and vegetables. Some parents buy special baby food recipe books and make exotic concoctions while others keep it much more simple.

All of these options can work for babies whether they are orally fed or tube fed.

There is a continuum and range of food preparation choices that parents make in feeding their families. These choices are mirrored in the choices which are made in preparing homemade blended formula for tube feeding.

Some families move from baby formula to commercially available purees, to a graded sequence of commercially prepared baby food, to commercially prepared toddler dinners, to family foods. Others provide breast milk for as long as possible and then offer blended or mashed fresh foods and never use commercial baby foods. Some very busy families tend to eat pre-packaged meals and fast foods. They often select a family restaurant to reduce the time and energy needed to prepare their own meals. Other parents enjoy taking the same amount of time to prepare family meals in crock-pots, filling the home with smells of slowly cooking foods that are ready to serve at the end of the workday. Many families prepare meals that include a combination of some prepared and some homemade foods.

The continuum from commercially prepared foods to fresh food meals prepared at home (i.e. "from scratch" foods), also is seen in homemade blended formula meal choices. Most families start tube feeding supplementation with breast milk or a prescribed formula. Some transition to a commercial formula made from whole foods (such as Compleat® Pediatric by Novartis). Others tiptoe in the direction of a homemade blended formula by introducing one commercial baby food fruit or vegetable at a time.

As the child accepts each food, new foods are introduced until the child can digest a variety of baby foods. Many families work out a recipe for feeding bolus meals that are simply a combination of commercial baby foods and formula. Other families introduce baby foods first, and when the

child's digestive system seems to be handling a variety of basic foods, they shift to a puree of fresh fruits, vegetables, grains and high-protein sources for their tube feeding meals. Families may choose to prepare roasts, and blend them in a good blender rather than offer commercial baby food meats. Or they may choose to offer organic green beans rather than a commercial baby food or canned green bean option. It's a matter of family preference and personal choice.

Time Continuum

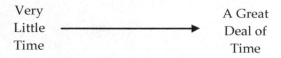

Very Little Time ————————————→ A Great Deal of Time

The amount of time needed to prepare family meals varies from a lot to very little. Time commitment is influenced by food choice, type of preparation, complexity of the menu and family schedule. On busy days, a restaurant meal, fast food or packaged prepared meal may be chosen. On other days, there's time to prepare a homemade meal with an exotic recipe. Meal preparation times vary from family to family, child to child and day to day for both orally fed and tube fed children.

The time needed to prepare a homemade blended formula is the choice of the preparer. Clearly, a blended diet made entirely out of recipe variations

of commercial baby foods requires a smaller preparation time commitment. This option is the first choice of many families. Other families may choose to combine fresh ingredients, roasted meats, and special herbs and spices to blend a recipe "from scratch." This choice, obviously, requires a greater time commitment.

Meal preparation time is a factor when meals are eaten away from home. When traveling, families may choose easier, quicker foods for tube meals such as a baby food blend or a prepackaged meal such as Real Food Blends. Commercial formulas, baby foods or a combination may be easier when staying at a hotel or on a family camping trip.

Cost Continuum

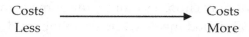

Costs Less ————————————→ Costs More

Like oral meals, tube meal costs vary along a continuum from less to more. Costs also vary with circumstances. Some insurance companies and health care systems pay for formula for tube fed children. Other families must pay out of pocket. This factor certainly influences decision making for many families. As with oral diets, tube food choices dictate meal costs. Commercial baby food peas may cost more than homemade blended frozen peas, and organically grown pea pods from a specialty store may cost even more per serving. Each family weighs the costs, time and value preferences in their decision making.

Time and cost are separate but related continuum scales when making homemade blended formulas. Sometimes we may prioritize cutting costs, even though it may take more time to prepare the formula. Other times, time is the most important aspect and we're willing to pay somewhat more for the convenience of prepared foods.

Practical Use of the Continuum Concept

Each continuum describes a process and series of choices. They're not meant to be a hierarchy in which parents move linearly from one to the other. Each choice is practical in terms of individual circumstances and preferences.

Parents can move in and out and slide back and forth on each continuum, depending on the circumstances of their child and family.

Clearly, a family will help a child move more linearly along a continuum when first introducing new foods into the diet. If the child handles the new food, it will be added to the diet and another new food will be tried. If the child does not tolerate it, the food will be eliminated (possibly to be tried again later), and another food will be introduced.

A wide variety of formulas and formula variations may be used, even within a single family. A child may be on a diet of three bolus meals a day of blended fresh foods, but the parent may choose to substitute some commercial baby food meals while traveling, or during a busy period. A child on a blended food diet may be given a very easily digested commercial formula for a few meals or a few days during an illness, depending on the child's digestive and health needs.

We describe movement on the continuum as simply that, "movement." It follows the child's lead and the family preferences. It's not intended to suggest that movement in one direction or another is "better" or "worse."

Homemade blended formulas are all about options – options that work for children and families. It's not about judgments and "shoulds." Working with their child's medical team, gaining knowledge of healthy diets, and trusting their hearts, parents can follow their children's lead to be wherever they need to be on each continuum.

For additional information on making decisions to explore a homemade blended formula diet see:

Klein, M.D. and Morris, S.E. (2007). Chapter 33 – Supporting Parents Who Choose a Homemade Blended Formula. *Homemade Blended Formula Handbook.* Tucson, AZ: Mealtime Notions, LLC

Real Food Blends
www.realfoodblends.com

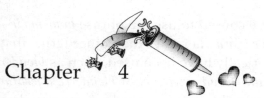

Our Perceptions of Mealtimes—
The Language We Choose

Chapter 4

Suzanne Evans Morris, Ph.D, CCC

We live in a world of verbal communication in which thoughts, beliefs and intentions are expressed through words. The words we use to describe a specific thought or situation are very important, for they can actually shift our perceptions of the event.

Think for a moment about some common phrases that we frequently encounter. When we talk about the *war on drugs* or the *fight against cancer,* we begin to think in a more aggressive or adversarial fashion about drugs or cancer. The language itself suggests that the only way to change the situation is to perceive drugs and cancer as enemies that we must battle. Could we be even more effective in our intention to reduce the problems of drugs in our society or to recover from cancer if we used a more peaceful set of words to express this desire? Perhaps we could speak of a *movement to reduce drug use* or *healing from cancer.* These alternative phrases invite more of a partnership in addressing the perceived problem, while maintaining a strong intention to change the situation.

Let's look at the language used to describe eating and consider the shifts in perception that might be experienced when different vocabulary is used to describe the same event.

Reflect on the differences in your perceptions and feelings if your *evening meal* were called your *evening feeding.* How might a child perceive receiving food in the morning if the process would be referred to as *breakfast* rather than the *morning tube feeding*?

Language choices can be empowering or disempowering for children and adults. When children are described as having a *feeding aversion* or *feeding resistance,* the focus is on the internal or external conflict with food or the persons offering the food.

The same youngsters could be described as *being worried or fearful about eating.* We could say that some children are *reluctant to eat because they haven't had many positive experiences around food.* A baby might be *pushing away because he doesn't trust that food will feel comfortable in his tummy.*

These words and descriptions enable us to focus attention on the factors that are influencing these children's responses to food and mealtimes (i.e. fear, worry, lack of positive experiences, lack of trust). They empower parents and professionals to focus on interactions during the mealtime that invite participation rather than resistance. They empower children to take small steps toward greater comfort, confidence and trust because they feel the support of adults who understand what they're experiencing inside and are willing to help them become more comfortable.

Our preference is to use the term *mealtimes* in all references to the child's interaction with food. *Mealtimes* invite participation and interaction with the child who is receiving food. *Feedings* create a more passive image, in which the child is less of a partner in the process.

Families will consciously find the vocabulary that's meaningful to them. Some make a descriptive distinction between food taken by tube and food taken by mouth. They may refer to their child's *mouth meals, oral meals, tasting meals* or *chewy meals.* These are contrasted with *tube meals, pump meals,* or *tummy meals.* Others will describe the specific meal as they would with children who are fed orally. The child simply gets *breakfast, morning snack, lunch, afternoon snack, dinner* or *supper.*

We want to create a vocabulary that celebrates the child's inclusion and participation in the family meal. We desire a language that focuses on the child's similarities to other children, not just the differences that often become the focus of our language and perception.

We also encourage parents and professionals to select words and ideas that reflect the home and family, and not the hospital and medical procedures. Historically there's been a gradual shift in which tube feedings have become a medical procedure. Many professionals and parents describe giving the child a *bolus, drip-feeding, pump feeding* or *syringe feeding*. Feeding-pump manufacturers refer to the amount of food as a *dose* of formula. These words create images of a medical environment rather than a home and family-friendly space in which people come together to eat.

The manner in which the child eats can be provided as an add-on description. Young children eat their cereal *with a spoon* or drink their milk *from a bottle*. Children who receive their nourishment through a tube could be described as eating their breakfast meal *through their tube* or getting their evening snack *from a feeding pump*.

We've chosen to use the phrase *homemade blended formula* rather than other terms that historically have been used, such as *blenderized formula, blenderized diet* or *blenderized feedings*. The term *homemade* is vitally important because it celebrates and honors the personal care and contributions that go into the formula. The term reflects a sharing of personal nurturing along with the nourishing foods the child needs to grow and be healthy.

Some families call this a *homemade blended meal*. Within the home, this term accurately reflects both the intention and the content of the food that's given. However, we decided to include the word *formula*, even though it's a more scientific term. In the broader experience of professionals and parents, we felt that *homemade blended formula* helped to differentiate the more liquid blended meals provided by tube from the blended pureed meals or soups given to individuals who eat orally.

For additional information on tube feeding mealtime concepts see:

Tannen, D. (1999). *The Argument Culture: Moving from Debate to Dialogue.* New York, NY: Ballantine Books.

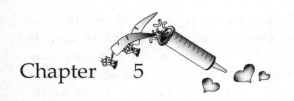

Chapter 5

Why Homemade Formulas?

Suzanne Evans Morris, Ph.D, CCC

Parents are frequently asked why they even would consider trying to make their own formula.

Professionals point out the nutritional consistency and ease of using a formula designed for children receiving tube feedings. Other parents comment that their lives are already so busy that it's a relief not to have to think about making a special meal for their child.

Yet every child and family is different, and a single nutritional solution doesn't fit everyone. Despite the differences among commercial formulas that allow for some fine tuning in children's dietary needs, these specialized formulas are limited in the choices they offer.

Through personal contact, sharing on Internet listservs and participation in several informal questionnaires, many parents have shared their perceptions, the reasons behind their choice of a homemade blended formula, and their child's responses to the formula changes. They've described the following advantages and benefits for themselves and their child of using a homemade formula:

- Parents feel more connected to their child's mealtimes because they're actively involved in preparing the meals.

- Parents feel more able to offer love through the food they prepare.

- Creating a homemade blended formula for their child provides emotional support for many parents who are grieving the loss of normal oral meals.

- Parents feel that they have more natural control in making choices about their child's diet when they're preparing the meals themselves.

- Children can participate in preparing their blended formula and feel more emotionally supported.

- Because children are receiving foods similar to what others are eating, parents recognize they are more similar to children who eat orally.

- Children can receive much greater dietary diversity in a homemade blended formula. This can make it easier for the child to accept new foods that are offered orally.

- Homemade blended formulas can contain many micronutrients that are only present in fresh fruits and vegetables. These phytonutrients are not present in processed formulas.

- Nutritious homemade blended formulas can cost less per meal than specialized tube feeding formulas. This represents a cost savings that can be very important for many families.

Feedback from Parents—Nourishing Themselves and Their Children

"I feel a greater sense of fulfillment through preparing my food for my baby, in my way. The whole process, from shopping for food, growing it (we grow most of our own vegetables), preparing it and cooking it is so important for a parent, I think. Parents of tube fed children miss out on so much feedback from their children and have to jump over so many natural stages in order to reach the stage that other parents are at, that it's nice to find a way to take back that natural process as much as we can. I think it has improved my relationship with my daughter more than I consciously realize - to be perfectly honest - it makes me see her as more 'normal' and more of a part of the family. Tube fed children 'eat'

too, they just do it through a tube. It's a bit like that. She eats proper food with us that we provide and prepare. She is not simply getting her stomach filled with formula from the pharmacy."

Jane

"I feel like I am doing something 'good' for her; I'm able to choose the ingredients, and often go with organic preparations, even though I don't feed the rest of the family organic. I feel good in doing this, I think partly because I completely breast-fed my other two kids and was heartbroken after five weeks of my daughter's life when it was obvious that she was not thriving on breast milk and was not interested in eating orally at all. A nasogastric tube was placed and we pumped high calorie formula into it. Eventually she needed the more permanent g-tube button as she developed a total oral and feeding aversion. I hated using the formulas. I hated that I couldn't even pronounce most of the ingredients on the label and wondered what synthetic substances I was feeding her. The homemade blended diet makes me feel much better, and gives me peace of mind. Logically, I know the commercial formulas are 'complete' foods, but psychologically I am so against them, maybe because I was a breast-feeding mom to start with."

Pam

"From a mom's perspective, I feel that I'm providing my son more of what he needs to grow. I'm less concerned now with him getting enough protein or nutrients than when I was relying on a can of formula. I also see the difference in my child that makes me know that the time it takes to prepare is worth every moment of it."

Kim

"I loved the feeling I was giving my child REAL foods and not a chemical concoction. Parent have a deep instinctual need to 'feed' their child and this was more satisfying to that need for me than processed formulas."

Rose-Marie

The homemade blended diets offered by parents differ substantially in the exact content of the formula and in the way it's introduced and then fine-tuned to the child's needs. Homemade blended formulas affect every child differently.

When changes are made slowly and in consultation with the child's medical team, and then introduced into a nurturing, communicative environment, many families have noticed the following responses of their children. Responses were unique to each child and not all children showed observable changes when receiving a homemade blended formula. We can only hypothesize about the reasons why some of these changes occurred.

Some Parents Tell Us That Their Children...

Change	Possible Reason
. . . increased the amount of formula they could take comfortably at one time.	Less gastrointestinal distress would lead toward a comfortable increase in volume.
. . . gained weight, while taking the same or fewer calories. Many of these children had not grown well on the commercial formula.	The homemade formula may have provided additional nutrients that the body needed to digest the food and utilize the calories. A reduction in stress at mealtimes may have reduced the fight-or-flight protective responses of the body and shifted it toward improved growth.

Some Parents Tell Us That Their Children...

Change	Possible Reason
. . . experienced less reflux, vomiting, gagging and retching. Testing showed that some children no longer had reflux.	Varying the foods in the formula and emphasizing dietary diversity can reduce allergic sensitivity to foods that are eaten on a daily basis. The heavier homemade formula stays in the stomach more easily than a thin, light formula. Formulas that are high in sugar content can be irritating to the entire digestive system for some children.
. . . had improved efficiency of digestion. There was more rapid gastric emptying and fewer smelly bowel movements.	Foods selected to be more compatible with the individual child's body can create less stress. Gastric emptying time is typically improved when there is less stress at mealtimes. Some parents added probiotics and digestive enzymes to the formula, which would have assisted efficient digestion
. . . showed improved bowel function and problems with constipation and diarrhea resolved.	Foods selected for a homemade blended formula typically contain more fiber than commercial formulas. Parents of toddlers and children often add additional water between meals.
. . . had less drooling and mucus production and medications to reduce mucus were discontinued	The body produces more mucus and saliva to protect the esophagus from acid reflux. If the homemade formula contributes to better digestion and less reflux, the body may no longer need the added mucus to protect its tissues
. . . had a better appetite and were interested in eating more food by mouth.	When children feel better, they're more interested in eating. Reducing or eliminating reflux helps many children become aware of more subtle hunger signals for the first time.
. . . were more interested in tasting and eating foods orally that they had first experienced through the tube	Children receive smell and taste sensations from food that is burped or in other ways enters the air stream that comes up the esophagus. They are more familiar with these foods and are more likely to develop an interest in exploring them by mouth.
. . . felt better and showed more interest in learning and participating in activities. Some children had better color and were more robust. Their energy level was higher.	Many components of a homemade blended formula can contribute to greater health and physical and emotional well being. Powerful blenders break down food fibers more efficiently, releasing nutrients more fully.

Changes are more likely to occur when parents take time to observe, interpret and follow their child's cues.

A dietitian typically creates an initial formula with a combination of foods and a schedule that makes sense nutritionally. Parents introduce changes slowly and systematically in a nurturing environment. They rely on verbal or nonverbal feedback from their children to guide them. If the homemade blended diet works, they continue it. If it doesn't work, they ask "why not" and make modifications. The child is the one who tells us about the appropriateness of the dietary choices, the volume and the pace of feeding. This is the pattern followed by orally fed children.

Feedback from Parents about Changes Through Homemade Blended Formulas

"She enjoys helping make it. She's able to tell me what she would like to have and she's able to build a happy relationship with food, which is the stepping stone to feeding therapy. I firmly believe her wonderful growth spurt in the past six months is due to the real food added to her diet."

Tawnia

"Physically, she is now above the 50th percentile for weight and the 75th for height. I have lost count of how many professional people have said she doesn't look like a tube fed child. She is extremely healthy and throws off infections and viruses easily now."

Jane

"Within two days of using my 'final recipe' blended diet, she ceased to retch and gag during her feedings, which she did for almost two years of feeding her various hypoallergenic formulas at different rates and volumes, with different reflux meds and combinations of meds. Coincidence? I don't think so. She is now showing interest in putting foods in her mouth, for the first time ever. I am confident that one day she will be an oral eater and I believe it is because she no longer retches and gags during her tube feedings."

Pam

"He looks healthier, has less reflux, and is less pasty looking."

Laura

"There is much less gagging and retching. While it is not eliminated, it is an incredible difference. My son used to cry for an hour after a tube feeding; now after a blended diet feeding he will get up and start moving once again."

Kim

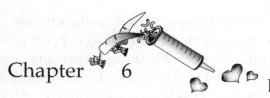

A Dietitian's Perspective on Homemade Blended Formulas

Chapter 6

Ellen Duperret, R.D., and Jude Trautlein, R.D.

As dietitians, we're meeting more and more families asking about a homemade blended formula. Can they provide it for their tube fed child? Where would they start? What should they put in the tube? How can they be sure they are putting in enough of the right kind of foods?

This has been a dilemma for dietitians. We've been taught that everything a child needs nutritionally is provided in commercially prepared formulas. Why would parents want to do anything different? These questions have forced us to look historically at tube feeding practices and to investigate the possibility of supporting these families. The fact is, many families feel very strongly about nourishing their children with their own homemade blend. We need to take these questions seriously and determine the best ways to support them.

Prior to the development of commercial formulas for tube feedings, families used homemade blenderized feedings, and in many countries of the world blending food for the tube is the standard practice even today. Commercial formulas first appeared in the 1950s, with more modern formulas appearing in the 1970s. The advantage of commercial formulas is that they're nutritionally complete with regard to vitamins, minerals, proteins, carbohydrates and fats. They're calorie-dense, with most supplying one calorie per ml for children over a year of age. They're easy for families and dietitians to quantify. Commercial formulas are safe in terms of food-borne illness, if they're handled properly after the cans are opened. They're convenient; families can simply open the can and pour it right into the tube feeding bag or syringe. And finally, commercial formulas are easy to use when families are away from home or traveling. These formulas revolutionized the tube feeding practices in the United States.

For all the above reasons, commercial formulas have worked well and continue to work well for many families. However, some parents today want to be able to prepare home cooked meals for their child and provide a more varied diet. They want to feed their tube fed child in a way more similar to the way they feed their other children. For families with the desire, time and resources needed to prepare homemade blended formulas, the move away from commercial formulas is an option.

Families who are successfully providing homemade blended formulas report a variety of positive changes in their children. Many families report a decrease in gagging, retching and vomiting. Bowel function improves, with many children no longer having constipation and no longer needing stool softeners. Those with chronically loose stools change to a more bulky formed stool. Many families state their children's stomachs seem more comfortable during and after a bolus of homemade formula. Families report that their children have less reflux and better stomach emptying. Other positive statements include that their children seem to get sick less frequently and have less mucous production. Families say their children are more willing to try oral food after starting homemade formula.

Additionally, tube fed children can help with food preparation and blending of homemade blended formulas, which gives them a more active role in the whole process. And finally, parents have felt pleased that they can provide a very healthy diet with a homemade blended formula, adding a variety of fruits and vegetables and other nutritious foods that children their age without tubes are often unwilling to eat. We kept hearing these positive statements and couldn't help but be impressed.

We've supported many families in their journey towards homemade blended formulas. Initially we, and many other health care professionals, had limited experience, but we were committed to learn. We learned from families who successfully added blended foods to their child's diet. We learned by asking questions of medical teams. We learned by making this journey with families, monitoring responses to the blended foods, analyzing diets, and watching growth.

Our approach to helping families move toward a homemade blended formula includes:

- Checking with the medical team to fully understand the child's dietary needs and restrictions.

- Starting slowly, making one change at a time and watching the child's response.

- Making sure parents fully understand the need for good food preparation, storage and hygiene.

- Carefully monitoring growth.

- Regularly analyzing the diet to insure optimum overall nutrients.

- Monitoring hydration.

- Learning from each family and each child. We've also provided tube feeding support groups for families interested in using homemade blended formulas. These have been offered with two dietitians, a feeding specialist and a pediatrician. We meet with families providing homemade blended formulas on a monthly basis. Parents and professionals share how things are going – what's working and what's not. It's been a tremendous support for families. We suggest it as an excellent way for professionals with limited homemade blended formula experience to see the benefits and fine-tune the process.

Homemade blended formulas are certainly not for everyone. However, as dietitians we can no longer say "no" to everyone who asks simply because our only experience has been with commercial formulas. We need to consider the possibility, ask good questions and work with each family on an individual basis to determine what works best for that child.

With any tube feeding it's important to get the support of a registered dietitian.

For more information on the dietitians approach to homemade blended formulas see:

> Duperret, E., Trautlein. J. & Klein, M.D. (2004). Homemade Blenderized Formula. *Nutrition Focus*, 19:5.

For additional information on the history of tube feedings see:

> Harkness, L. (2002). The History of Enteral Nutrition Therapy: From Raw Eggs and Nasal Tubes to Purified Amino Acids and Early Postoperative Jejunal Delivery. *Journal American Dietetic Association*, 102:3, 399-404.

A Pediatrician's Perspective on Homemade Blended Formulas

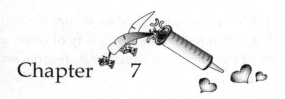

Chapter 7

Sanford Newmark, M.D.

Why would a pediatrician be interested in seeing tube fed infants and children switched from a commercial formula to a blended homemade formula made from real foods? There are a number of good reasons, but before I discuss these, let me reverse the question. Would any pediatrician encourage orally fed children who are over 6 to 9 months old to be fed exclusively by commercial formula?

As pediatricians, we encourage the introduction of solid foods by 4 to 6 months, and would be very concerned about, for example, an 18-month-old who is not taking any solid foods. Most tube fed children are not tube fed because they have different nutritional needs from other children, but because they're unable to take orally the foods they need, due to neurological, gastrointestinal, or sometimes psychosocial issues. Therefore, they have the same nutritional need for whole foods that most other children have. I believe these children should be exclusively fed a commercial formula only if there is some good medical reason not to give them whole foods.

Before discussing the many advantages of whole foods though, I'd like to acknowledge that there are valid reasons why some parents may not be able to undertake the very significant commitment that providing a totally homemade blended formula entails. These reasons often involve the lack of time, energy and resources that are common in our society in general and especially for those caring for a child with special needs. Later in this chapter, I'll make some suggestions for those parents who are interested but not currently able to make the complete switch.

Missing Ingredients

The most crucial reason I support homemade formulas is that I do not believe commercial formulas provide all the essential nutrients that whole foods do. Of course, they provide the basic protein, fat, carbohydrates and vitamins necessary for growth, but they're missing other nutrients we know are crucial to optimal health and development, and some we may not yet have discovered.

What are these missing items? One very good example is Omega-3 fatty acids. We know that DHA, one of the Omega-3 fatty acids, is very important to normal neurological development. This is so widely accepted by the scientific community that it has been added to many pre-term and term infant formulas (such as Lipil®). One recent research study showed that premature infants fed formula with DHA had better intellectual and motor development at two years old than infants not given extra DHA. Yet, as of this printing, there is still no significant amount of DHA or Omega-3 Fatty Acids in some commercial formulas for children over a year old. This is even more important because many tube fed infants also have developmental delays and need all the neurological, intellectual and motor encouragement they can get.

Another example of nutrients provided in insufficient quantity in commercial formulas is the phytonutrients that are available from many fruits and vegetables. Phytonutrients are compounds that have powerful antioxidant (and other) beneficial effects, but are not vitamins. Just a partial list of these phytonutrients includes flavonoids, carotenoids, isoflavones and phenols. We are continually discovering more information about the number and importance of these compounds as nutritional research progresses. These are probably responsible for the fact that an increased intake of fruits and vegetables definitely leads to a decreased risk of cancer, and the availability of phytonutrients is one of the main reasons the National Cancer Institute recommends five to nine servings of fruits and vegetables per day. Commercial formulas don't provide any of these recommended phytonutrients. Therefore, they should be added to the diets of tube fed children receiving only commercial formula.

Scientific research is continually discovering substances in food that are responsible for optimal health and development. We constantly see research articles and nutritional updates about the newest nutrient we should include in our diets. Food nutrients work together like a finely tuned symphony. Science may be able to identify a few of the players, but as yet lacks knowledge and understanding of how all the ingredients in whole foods work together. Adding single nutrients as a supplement to commercial formulas has limited value because we don't have the whole picture of how they fit in with other nutrients in food, many of which haven't even been identified. That's why it's so necessary to feed children a varied diet with adequate amounts of the various food groups, whether by mouth or feeding tube. There are a number of research studies indicating that dietary diversity in itself may be associated with more positive health outcomes.

The bottom line, then, is that even if we were to supplement commercial formulas with all the elements we knew were missing from them, we would very likely still be missing some nutrients essential for our children's optimal health.

Influence on Oral Feeding

Another reason that I encourage the use of blended homemade formulas is that I believe their use increases the likelihood of successful oral feeding. I've talked to a number of parents who found their tube fed children who were taking some oral foods began to take in more by mouth when they were switched to homemade blended foods. This makes sense from a scientific point of view. After all, all of the flavors from foods placed into the gastrostomy tube are absorbed into the bloodstream, and these influence children's perception of taste. It's well-known by parents, pediatricians, and dietitians that one often has to

offer babies a food several times before they enjoy eating it. Blenderized food is a way of offering a variety of food tastes to babies and children on a regular basis.

We even know that foods that mothers eat during pregnancy and breastfeeding influence how much a baby will enjoy certain foods. In one study, mothers were given carrot juice during pregnancy and their babies had a more positive reaction to carrot juice when it was first offered. The same was true if the mothers drank carrot juice while breastfeeding. So it's not hard to understand why exposing children to a wide variety of healthful foods through the tube could lead to a positive impact on current and future oral feeding behavior.

Intestinal Influences

A common complication of commercial formula is called "dumping syndrome." This occurs when liquid formula is so quickly absorbed by the small intestine that it leads to a sharp increase in blood sugar, followed by an insulin spike, and then a sharp decrease in blood sugar causing hypo-glycemia and a number of other problems. This is mainly caused by the fact that most of the carbohydrate in commercial formula has been processed and broken down into more simple sugars. Using cornstarch to decrease the rate of absorption of sugar can sometimes successfully treat the problem, but it's not an ideal solution. I'm also very suspicious that many children have subtler effects of being fed only highly processed carbohydrates, without having an overt dumping syndrome. We know that for healthy children, eating complex unprocessed carbohydrates is much more healthful than eating processed carbohydrates, so why shouldn't this be true of tube fed children? One of my recent patients had her dumping syndrome completely resolve after she made the gradual switch from formula to foods. Fiber also helps decrease the rate of sugar absorption so when parents are using a com-mercial formula, it may be more effective to select one with added fiber.

Slow gastric emptying is a common problem in tube fed infants. Formula remains in the stomach for a long time and interferes with the total amount of food that a child can take at a meal. Many children are uncomfortable and limit the number of ounces of formula they eat at lunch because a substantial portion of breakfast is still in their stomachs. This can cause difficulty with supplying enough calories, and increases the likelihood of reflux symptoms. It's not totally clear how using a homemade blended formula would affect this problem. Thickened feedings do seem to prevent reflux in some children. One study showed they increased the rate of gastric emptying. However, fiber can slightly decrease the rate of gastric emptying.

Reducing Stress

Additionally, it's been shown that stress decreases gastric emptying. When humans are stressed, they produce a hormone named corticotrophin releasing factor, which leads to both an increase in the time it takes for the stomach to empty and an increase in the sensitivity of the gastrointestinal system in general. Therefore, an important part of the approach to tube feeding includes having the least stressful mealtimes possible, for both parents and children.

As an integrative physician, I believe that one has to consider not only the body, but also the mind and emotions of each child. Further, children must be seen not just as separate individuals, but also in relationship to their families and communities. In the case of tube feeding, we need to consider not only the nutritional factors involved, but also the child's and parents' mental and emotional relationships to feeding. For instance, a tube fed five year old may benefit greatly from the empowerment of choosing some of what goes into his or her tube, and this may improve future chances of developing good oral feeding skills.

On the other hand, if a working single mother becomes upset and stressed at the difficulty of preparing a total homemade blended formula for her 9-month-old, he or she could easily pick up this stress, resulting in poorer digestion and perhaps increased gastrointestinal discomfort.

From the viewpoint of parent-child bonding and satisfaction with the feeding process, I again think a homemade blended formula has certain advantages. Tube feeding time is still a mealtime, and can give much of the satisfaction that parents and children find in normal mealtimes. I think that for some mothers and fathers the selection of healthful, wholesome foods is a joyful and important part of the parenting process, and this can be just as rewarding when developing a diet for the tube fed child. For those parents with the time and resources, the buying, selecting and preparing of their child's food can be a wonderful away of expressing commitment and love.

Food Sensitivities

Another area that concerns me about commercial formula is the development of food sensitivities. When a child is given a single formula as the only source of nutrition, it seems to me that there is a higher likelihood of developing food sensitivities. I've seen a number of children who were given milk-based formulas by gastrostomy tube who developed chronic problems like constipation, reflux, irritability, and poor sleep that resolved after the formula was changed. Of course, one could make the argument that the solution would be a hypoallergenic formula with no milk protein. However, these formulas are very expensive and it makes more sense to avoid the problem by giving a varied and whole-food-based diet as soon as possible.

The Continuum

What would I recommend for those parents unable to make the complete switch to homemade blended formula? I think this can be seen as a process and as part of a continuum. Perhaps parents could add a single jar of baby food to the formula three times a day. I also strongly recommend adding an Omega-3 supplement to the formula. This is fairly easy, need not be expensive, and is a good choice for those who don't have time to create a formula that includes foods with high levels of Omega-3s. There also are some multivitamin and mineral supplements that include some of the added phytonutrients that are so healthful for children.

It's extremely important to work with a dietitian or a pediatrician when making these types of dietary changes or additions for a tube fed child, to ensure the child doesn't get too much of any single vitamin, because there are vitamins in the formulas. There are even some supplements that consist of dried fruits and vegetables in a powdered form, which might be the next best thing to blending fruits and vegetables for the tube feeding formula.

It's important to remember that some children have more complex nutritional problems. Multiple food allergies, celiac disease, mal-absorption syndromes and metabolic problems can make feeding certain children orally or by tube very complex task. However, this doesn't mean that feeding a homemade blended formula is impossible. It simply means that it will need to be done with even closer cooperation between the pediatrician, dietitian and other specialists.

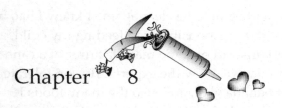

Chapter 8

A Parent's Perspective: Nourishing and Nurturing

Trish Whitehouse

My son Bobby was born with a congenital heart defect requiring a series of surgeries, the first at four days of age.

That first surgery went well and Bobby came home in 10 days with a nasogastric tube down his nose. Because he was a bit of a preemie (4 lbs) and weak from the surgery, I, being a nurse, convinced the hospital staff to discharge him with the feeding tube so that feeding issues wouldn't delay our discharge. Over the next three months, he transitioned off the nasogastric tube onto total breastfeeding.

Bobby went in for his second surgery at 3 months old, but this time things didn't go as smoothly and he ended up in intensive care for the next three months. He had every possible intervention to keep him alive. There were numerous tubes down his throat so he could be hooked up to a breathing machine, chest tubes, IV and monitoring lines, suctioning down his throat on an hourly basis, tubes up his nose, on his face and everywhere there was an available patch of open skin.

When Bobby came home from the hospital the second time, he wouldn't let anything in his mouth. I was told it was an aversion, or fear, because he had had so much inserted down his throat against his will. This caused him to be fearful that something else near his mouth or throat was just going to cause more pain. His muscle tone was atrocious; he looked like a limp dishrag, couldn't lift his head and his abdominal muscles were very weak. I was told that this aggravated his reflux and made him even more reluctant to eat. Also, because he had been intubated so many times, his gag reflex moved from the back of his throat to the front of his tongue, so whenever anything hit the front of his mouth, he'd just throw up.

If there was one thing about raising babies that I *knew* how to do, it was feed them. I had nursed three children who followed a nice steady curve on the growth charts as they reached all the crucial milestones. I loved breastfeeding my children, attending every breastfeeding conference I could find to learn more and providing peer counseling to other breast-feeding mothers. I had hopes of augmenting my nursing degree with a lactation consultant certification and thought I didn't have much of anything else to learn about how to help a newborn thrive.

So when I was told that I could not breastfeed my child and that he was intolerant of the fat in my milk because of a complication that occurred during his cardiac surgery, it was as if someone had just taken my last shred of parental control and thrown it to the wind. I felt like I got kicked in the stomach.

Having a child with a feeding tube, for me, was the ultimate insult. As a competent nursing mother, I had learned to nurture, console, quiet, comfort, feed and mostly love my children by breastfeeding. It wasn't just a form of food, it was a way of life for me. It was a means to an intimacy and bonding with my children that I'd never dreamed of before my babies were born. To have that taken away, and replaced with a silicone feeding tube, feeding pump, numbers, measurements, times, amounts and food from a can, was akin to taking away my role as a mother and totally overriding my instincts…those instincts that I had spent 12 years refining and honoring in myself… those same instincts that I used to define who I was.

I knew I had to pump my milk for my baby. The complication requiring non-fat milk was temporary and when Bobby again could have full-fat breast milk, I pumped around the clock for him, just as I would have nursed my other infants. But breastfeeding is much more than just food, so I had to find other ways to substitute for the things breastfeeding could do.

For example, many times my babies fell asleep cuddling and suckling at my breast. That was the most difficult aspect of not being able to nurse Bobby -- now I didn't have those easy means of comfort available to me. So at night I used to put him in a sling-type carrier and pace the living room floor, back and forth, over and over, while I pushed the vacuum around for the white noise, with the feeding pump bag slung over my shoulder giving him continuous nutrition, all the while singing lullabies to my drowsy son. Although it wasn't a cuddly baby nursing to sleep, it was the best I could do. Often I would take my shirt off to give him the skin-on-skin closeness I knew babies thrive on so well during those first few weeks.

I pumped my milk for a very long time to provide it as his sole source of nutrition, and it was heartbreaking to me when my son would projectile vomit all the precious milk it had taken me so long to pump. But I kept pumping because it gave me a purpose and a role in my son's nutrition.

When Bobby was old enough, I began to feed him blended foods through his tube. I clearly remember the first time I put real food through his tube as being one of the happiest days since he got the feeding tube.

With my other three children, I remember taking great pride in mashing up that first banana and putting it up to their lips, anticipating what they would do with it and how they would accept this first taste of something other than breast milk. Sometimes they were eager to try more, but most often they just played with it and made faces. Bobby did not want to play with food because it made him gag or vomit. When I mashed up that first banana to put through Bobby's tube and mixed it with my breast milk, I was even more excited than with my other three. My role as a

mother began to be clear again. I knew I had an important responsibility in feeding my child, and that I, instead of some manufacturer of a canned formula, was now the expert. My son tolerated that banana well, and also the many foods I introduced after that day. I was hooked on the idea of "real" food through the tube.

I began to get excited about going shopping, where before the thought of feeding my son depressed me. Now I went to the baby food aisle looking for ideas on what I could puree and feed my son through the tube. After a few months of introducing foods slowly, one by one, and allowing a period of time to go by to see if he reacted in any negative way, I had quite an array of foods to feed him.

I was actually having fun preparing his meals now and I fed him like I would have my other children. A little bit of cereal and breastmilk for breakfast, maybe a sandwich, some tofu and rice, fruit and a cookie for lunch, and a nice home cooked meal with vegetables, protein and carbohydrates for dinner. I didn't need to be a chemist, just a mother of four who used her common sense to feed her family healthy well-balanced meals. I put what I would have liked Bobby to eat by mouth on his high chair tray and, on a good day, he'd play with it. Then I'd put it in a blender with enough breast milk to thin it out and feed it to him through his tube.

Bobby immediately reacted favorably to his new diet. The first improvement was that his blood iron level rose significantly and we were able to stop his iron supplement. His hair grew in thicker with a shiny blond color. He had more energy, and went from barely sitting up by himself at the age of one year to crawling the very next month after starting blended foods. His stools were healthier and less runny. His reflux decreased dramatically.

But the best "improvement" from his real food diet was the change in his mother. I felt needed, intelligent, proud and like a mother again. My instincts, which had been so badly stifled because of having to feed my child through a tube, were finally allowed to surface and be acknowledged. I practically danced my way through the aisles of the grocery store, with my tube fed son and his optimal nutrition in the forefront of my mind. Not only could I love my son through my actions, but now I could show him I loved him through my food.

It might sound a little crazy—after all what does food have to do with love? But I think it's a vital component of every mother–child relationship. Feeding our children and watching them thrive is the very first thing we can do for our helpless infants. They depend on us to act in their behalf and listen to our instincts. We listen to them cry and realize they're hungry. We nuzzle them close when they're feeding, and we kiss their foreheads many times while they're being nourished. We bond, we enjoy, we communicate and we express our deepest love. That is all taken away when the act of feeding is mechanical, technical, intimidating and distant, as it can be with a feeding tube.

By blending Bobby's meals and giving him the same real food my other children had at his age, I felt really needed. Before this, it had seemed like the medical professionals were the real experts in his life, and that what I said and did really didn't matter. That may not have been true, but that's how it felt. It was as though my role in raising my own child had been replaced by modern medicine. After all, without their expertise, he wouldn't be alive, so what did my input matter?

But my input did matter. It mattered a lot. There was nothing that could replace my wisdom as a mother, and nothing insignificant about laughing and playing with Bobby to stimulate his brain development and social well being. And—though I sought assistance from my doctor on what to feed Bobby—no medical degree could improve my ability to nurture and love my child through his day to day feeding.

My son is now a 100% oral eater. In retrospect, I think Bobby's lack of interest in eating orally was probably a combination of many things, and what worked to allow him to eat by mouth probably was a combination as well.

Though I don't wish to go back to the tube feeding days, I do miss knowing that Bobby is getting those well-balanced, nutrient-dense meals he got when I used to grind up the family's favorites. My other children used to help me pick out what we'd feed Bobby through the tube, and they were always sure to give him a sweet treat at the end. I think that helped them see their little brother as a real person and not some machine we fed some of that "stuff" into.

It's easy to think that the tube doesn't affect the other children in the family, but I remember my five year old asking me one day, obviously concerned and very serious, "Mom, when am I going to have to have a tube?" But before I could reassure her that she probably would never need one, she continued, "...because he gets really good stuff through there!"

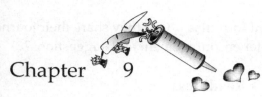

Chapter 9
Is a Homemade Blended Formula Right for You and Your Child?

Marsha Dunn Klein, M.Ed., OTR/L

Choosing to provide a homemade blended formula for your child is a personal decision based on information that only you, your physician, your dietitian and your child know.

First and foremost, remember that feeding is a relationship between parent and child. Ideally, it's a time of closeness that allows both parents and children to enjoy each other and build trust. It's a time of communication and understanding each other's cues. It's highly personal. What is right and works for one family is not necessarily what is right or what works for another.

Parents and children both bring information to the mealtime. Parents bring information about the techniques of tube feeding, diet, their experiences with mealtimes, their expectations, fears, confidence and beliefs. Children contribute information about their own bodies, what feels good and what doesn't and their perceptions of mealtimes based on past experiences. A homemade formula decision will be influenced by many of these factors.

Keeping "The Decision" in Perspective

Remember we consider a homemade blended formula to be ANY addition of pureed food to the commercial formula diet. We describe it as a continuum that ranges from as little as adding a bit of pureed fruit once daily to the formula, to as much as a complete diet of only homemade blended foods or family meals given through the feeding tube.

We're never sure when we add any new foods to a diet how the child will respond. It's a learning process for both parent and child. Will the child handle some additional puree and show improved results, or will the homemade puree in some way cause increased stress for the child? The decision to offer a homemade blended formula is essentially a choice to *explore* a new mealtime

possibility. This involves picking a food and starting slowly and carefully to see where that decision takes you. The decision does not involve using a commercial formula one day and transitioning the next day to a pre-decided "recipe" for a blended diet. By looking at the decision as merely a starting point rather than a final decision, many families and professionals are greatly relieved.

How are Things Going NOW?

Parents know themselves and their family best. They know how they're feeling about the commercial formula option. They know how well feedings are going now. Some families are eager to change what they feed their children. They're very upset with the commercial formula option and want support to make the change immediately. Other families feel accepting of commercial formulas and take more of an "if it's not broken don't fix it" attitude. For many families, the medical issues that lead up to the placement of the tube have been so complicated that they're relieved to have finally found a balance of calories, formula and volume that works for them and their child. Change is the last thing on their mind.

Support

Parents tell us they want support in providing homemade blended options. This frequently influences whether they'll decide to explore a homemade blended formula for their child. What type of support is available and how can they access it?

Is the pediatrician or family doctor open to the idea of a homemade blended formula? Physicians can help parents decide whether it's medically appropriate to introduce a non-commercial formula. Many physicians are new to the concept of homemade blended formulas. They can support

33

families by telling them honestly that they do not know if it will work well for their child, but that there may be no medical reasons why they cannot support your efforts to try it. For some children with highly specialized nutritional needs they may recommend staying with the commercial formula as the best medical option. They can be another set of eyes to look at the big picture of the feedings and help families determine a right time to explore moving toward a blended formula. Pediatricians can provide ongoing support when parents move in the direction of homemade blended formulas.

Is there a dietitian who can help the family make nutritional decisions, and look at recipes, nutrients and growth? Dietitians help families as they increase the amount and variety of pureed foods and try to balance quantities of formula with quantities of puree. They have the skills and experience to analyze recipes and help parents look at overall nutrients. Dietitions understand the big picture of growth.

Is there a feeding therapist who can help the family explore how to present the tube feedings in interactive ways that engage the child's ability to communicate comfort, discomfort, hunger, thirst and fullness during a meal? Parents often miss communication cues that can guide a meal because they haven't considered the subtle shifts of attention, facial expression and muscle tone that reflect the child's needs, wants and inner comfort. Feeding therapists can show families how to help their children make the connection between using their mouths and being hungry or full, and how to build the child's trust of the sensory and motor aspects of mealtimes.

Is there family support? Are both parents interested in exploring a blended formula? Just as parents of orally fed children need to work together to provide optimum nutrition for their child, parents of tube fed children need to work out details of a homemade blended formula together.

Is there support from other parents of tube fed children who have had success with homemade

blended formulas ? Can they share their journeys and offer encouragement and suggestions?

Child's Readiness

Is the child ready for a new formula? Physicians can give parents input regarding their child's readiness for dietary change. Many families try to find a time where tube feedings are as stable as possible. If the child is sick, vomiting constantly, and in any type of medical crisis, it is not the time to start a new diet. It is so important to watch a child's reaction to each new puree offered, and if the child is having wide fluctuations in physical reactions and is not feeling well when a new food is introduced, it is hard to know if a negative response is related to overall health issues or is a reaction to a particular food.

Sometimes families feel that the timing is not optimal to introduce a blended formula to their child right now. However, they may reconsider the option at another time when the child's overall health and feeding regime are more stable.

Parent Readiness

Many children who use a feeding tube have experienced complicated medical challenges. Family members often respond by feeling stressed to varying degrees. The amount of stress each individual feels varies with the nature of the medical complications and the personal experiences of both the child and parent. It is also highly dependent upon each person's perception of the experience. Two parents, for example, may experience the same external event, such as a surgery to place a feeding tube. The amount and type of stress, however, depends upon how individuals perceive tube feedings and whether or not they believe that the feeding tube is in the best interest of their child and family.

Changes in the daily routine can increase stress levels, especially when the parent cannot predict how the child will respond to a change in the mealtime routine. It is important for parents to ask themselves if they are really ready for a change. Do they have the energy to try something new? Do they have the time and energy to offer, observe and monitor a new feeding routine? Sometimes it is a good time to start a blended formula and sometimes, realistically, it's better to postpone changes until the family has time and energy to focus on the efforts involved in change.

Choices and Variations

There are many choices that families can make to find the best ways of creating a homemade blended formula which fits their needs and resources. Most of these options can be viewed on a continuum of complexity of food, preparation, time and cost. Parents considering the shift to a homemade blended formula can review these options in other sections of this manual.

Expectations

There are no guarantees with any diet for any child. Parents and professionals create a diet plan for the child, offer it, observe the child's responses and revise the plan as needed. Parents need to be clear on their own goals and expectations as they consider shifting to a blended food diet. For some parents, the goal is to improve bowel movements and hopefully decrease constipation medications. For others it ultimately is to blend the family meal

and offer it through the tube. Homemade blended formula variations have made changes for many children. Some changes are dramatic while others are subtler. The changes are individual and the pace at which the child handles formula changes is personal. As we have emphasized, parents need to decide whether they wish to start modifying or changing their child's current diet. If they decide that they wish to explore this option, they will come up with a plan, start the process and observe their child's responses to this step-by-step process. Some parents offer a homemade food or two and realize that their child did not handle it well. At this point they may decide that the family needs to go back to the old regimen and introduce pureed foods again later. Or they may sense that their child would have a more positive response if different foods were offered or if they considered changes in food volume, timing or presentation.

We began this chapter by asking "Is a homemade blended formula right for you and your child?" The answer requires a careful consideration of many factors. Each family and child makes the final decision with information and input provided by medical, nutritional, and therapy team members.

For additional information on making the decision to explore a homemade blended formula diet see:

Klein, M.D. and Morris, S.E. (2007). Chapter 3 – The Continuum Concept in Homemade Blended Formulas. *Homemade Blended Formula Handbook.* Tucson, AZ: Mealtime Notions, LLC.

Klein, M.D. and Morris, S.E. (2007). Chapter 18 – Beginning a Homemade Blended Formula. *Homemade Blended Formula Handbook.* Tucson, AZ: Mealtime Notions, LLC.

Klein, M.D. and Morris, S.E. (2007). Chapter 33 – Supporting Parents Who Choose a Homemade Blended Formula. *Homemade Blended Formula Handbook.* Tucson, AZ : Mealtime Notions, LLC.

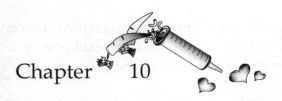

Chapter 10

Mealtime Communication and Homemade Blended Formulas

Suzanne Evans Morris, Ph.D, CCC

Mealtime communication offers the key to meals that are comfortable and nurturing to both child and parent.

As communicators, we play two distinct roles in any dialogue. We alternate between being the speaker and the listener. As the speaker we tell another person what we need or are thinking. As the listener we take in the information the speaker is sharing with us. We may act on that information or respond to it as we shift back to the role of speaker. The dialogue need not involve speech or words. It can occur entirely at the nonverbal level or with a mixture of verbal and nonverbal messages.

Our knowledge and ability to recognize and respond to messages from orally fed children provide a solid foundation for recognizing and responding to variations of the same messages which come from tube fed children.

When I offer my child sweet potatoes for dinner, this is a nonverbal communication in which my action of placing the food on the table is equivalent to saying, "Here are your sweet potatoes." I'm the initiator or speaker in this dialogue. My child can respond to this message in many different ways. She may move her body toward the food and smell it, as if to say, "I'm going to check out this funny orange stuff on my plate." She could pick up the spoon and open her mouth, nonverbally saying, "I'm ready for a bite of sweet potatoes." She might push the plate away and say "no food" to tell me she doesn't want it. She could eat a small amount and begin to squirm and look uncomfortable and say "all done." Her response in this situation could mean, "I'm hungry but I don't like the feeling of this food in my tummy. I'm uncomfortable," or "I'm really not hungry right now." Nonverbal babies and young children who are fed by mouth have many options for guiding the person feeding them.

They tell us "yes" by opening their mouths, making sucking movements and moving their bodies closer to the spoon and the person feeding them. They reach for the spoon or the bowl. They laugh and gurgle and make other happy noises. As they get older they tell us with words like "more milk" or "yummmy." They communicate "no" by turning their faces away, closing their mouths, moving away from the person feeding them and spitting out the food. They may frown or cry or tell us with words that they don't want the food or we're feeding them too fast and they're not ready for the next spoonful.

Some parents assume that if children don't speak or have very low cognitive abilities, they don't communicate. All living beings communicate. Communication occurs at many different levels. Vocalization and physical changes are the most basic signals that can be recognized as communicative signals. Newborns let us know when they're hungry, tired or stressed by different types of crying and by changing their breathing patterns and heart rate. Their skin color changes when they move from being comfortable to uncomfortable.

Most parents recognize and respond to their young infant's mealtime cues. There's an easy nonverbal conversation as the eager baby nuzzles into the mother's breast to receive milk and the mother responds by positioning her nipple so the infant can latch on easily. She recognizes the moments when her baby needs to be burped and the times when he simply wants to gaze into her eyes and be social. She responds appropriately.

Despite our natural programming to recognize a child's communication at mealtimes, parents and professionals often don't recognize these same messages when children receive a meal through a feeding tube.

It may take time to recognize the cues of a tube fed child, as they may be different from those of an orally fed child. This lack of recognition also may be related to our tendency to perceive tube feedings as a medical procedure that "must be done" rather than as a regular meal that happens to be given by a tube rather than a bottle or spoon.

Often, when tube fed children indicate they need a pause in the flow of the formula or are full and want to stop, adults fail to pay attention or override the early signals because there's still formula remaining in the pump or syringe. When the more subtle signals are ignored, children's discomfort and efforts to communicate escalate. At this point they may respond with major physiological signals of discomfort such as gagging, retching or vomiting. This scenario occurs infrequently when children are fed orally because they're rarely forced to eat more than they can handle comfortably.

The Division of Responsibility at Mealtimes

Parenting expert and dietitian, Ellyn Satter has described a division of responsibility at mealtimes that works well for families with children. These guidelines are just as applicable to children who receive meals through feeding tubes.

> Parents are responsible for *what*, *where* and *when* the child eats.
>
> Children are responsible for *how much* and *whether* they eat.

In this division of responsibility, adults select the foods that are served at the meal. They also decide where the meal will take place and the time of the meal. Their responsibility includes selecting nutritious foods that are appropriate to the child's age, sensory and physical abilities. Although the same basic foods are served to all members of the family, the toddler's food may be pureed or fork mashed while the older child may receive a more chewable version of the same foods. They decide whether the meal will take place at the kitchen table or during a picnic in the park. An early

dinner is more appropriate when there are very young children, while a later mealtime may suit older children and teenagers.

The parent's responsibility ends when the meal is placed on the table and food is offered to the child. At this point the child's responsibility begins. Children are the ones who decide which foods they'll eat and which ones they'll leave on the plate. They determine whether to eat one bite of peaches or the whole bowl. They discover new foods without adult pressure to eat them the first time they're served. Gradually the unfamiliar becomes more familiar and comfortable and new foods are added to the child's overall diet.

When these roles and responsibilities are honored, meals go smoothly. When the child takes over the parent's role or when the parent assumes the child's responsibility, problems arise.

Children may insist that their parents serve only foods that they like. If the adult selects carrots and chicken for lunch, they may pout and say that they don't like these foods and they won't eat them. They want macaroni and cheese! Many parents abdicate their responsibility for selecting the food and dutifully go to the kitchen to prepare a meal of macaroni for their child. The child may refuse to come to the table for dinner and will only eat when watching a favorite video. The whole family may end up eating in front of the television with the child instead of at the location chosen by the adult preparing the meal. Parents may give up on setting formal times for meals because their children eat whenever and whatever they want in a constant stream of child-directed snacks. Parents also take over areas that are their children's responsibility. They remind them to eat the carrots or tell them they can't leave the table until they finish the chicken. When the child says she's really full and is all done, the parent may tell her she has to drink all of her milk first.

In some cases adults don't fulfill their own responsibilities because they're spending all their time and energy taking care of their child's mealtime jobs. They may serve foods that are inappropriate for a youngster's skill level or that aggravate an allergy or reflux. They may offer meals in a location that's too over-stimulating or under-stimulating for their child. They may wait to feed a hungry toddler until older children come home from sports practice, and then find a little one who's too irritable to eat when the meal finally arrives.

Role reversals frequently lead to power contests, mealtime battles and even force-feeding, and parents become short-order cooks making a different meal for each family member. When adults decide how much food children must eat, children begin to ignore the internal commun-ication cues designed to match hunger levels with the amount of food eaten. Dietitians and doctors are beginning to recognize the role that this lack of awareness of inner cues plays in the increasing incidence of obesity in children.

Mealtime Communication and Tube Feeding

There's also a division of responsibility for tube meals. Parents still decide the what, where and when of tube feedings. Tube fed children let us know about the "how much" and whether the food choices we've made for them feel good in their tummies and help them grow!

When offering a child food through a tube, we need feedback about what's working and what's not. Is the food, amount and timing appropriate for the child? Without the child's feedback and our ability to recognize and interpret that feed-back, we can't do our part to create a homemade blended formula and offer it in a way that creates a comfortable eating experience.

We can become more observant during tube meals. As we become more aware of the child's facial expressions, vocalizations and mouth and body movements, we begin to see patterns, especially in relationship to the formula and the way we give it to the child.

For example, one mother noticed that when the meal was going well and her son was comfortable with the formula, he kicked his right leg rhythmically. He often made soft sounds and small sucking movements with his mouth. She observed that sometimes he pulled both legs up toward his abdomen and was very quiet. This was usually followed five minutes later by gagging and retching. She became aware that the only nonverbal mealtime signals she responded to were the stronger signals of discomfort at the end of this sequence. When he started to gag and retch, she stopped the flow of the formula and distracted him to prevent his vomiting. She realized that he often needed her to stop giving the formula when he was quiet for more than a minute. If he began to pull his legs up, she would place her hand on his abdomen and remind him to let go of the tightness in his tummy and take easy breaths to feel better.

Her son became more confident, experiencing less overall stress at mealtimes because he recognized that his mother was his communication partner. She listened, followed his lead and helped him.

His mother became more comfortable exploring small variations in the foods she used in the homemade blended formula, her timing in offering different amounts of the formula, and the total volume that her child could take at each meal. Her child's gagging, retching and vomiting stopped as they moved toward the mealtime alternatives which met his needs for comfort and interaction.

Children can use a wide variety of nonverbal signals to let us know where they are on the continuum from comfort to discomfort to distress. We're successful in interpreting "comfort" signs because everything is going well. The child is relaxed, calm, or happy. No change is demanded of us. We also are able to understand "distress" when the child is communicating at the extreme end of the continuum with blatant vomiting or gagging or crying.

It often takes parents a bit longer to understand some of the more subtle "discomfort" communications. Some children become serious and wide-eyed. Some produce more saliva and swallow more frequently when they're experiencing more reflux. Others purse their lips and make a sour face. Still others may rub their hair or pull on an ear or arch backwards to let us know they're beginning to feel uncomfortable.

Pauses are common during meals that children and adults eat orally. We take short breaks to talk to others, to enjoy the sensory input of the food and environment, and to respond to our inner signals of hunger or approaching fullness. It's interesting that this pattern of alternating periods of eating and short pauses has never become a recommended pattern for tube feeding meals. Perhaps regular or intermittent pauses should be considered.

A division of responsibility at mealtimes is appropriate for all children, including those who are tube fed. When parents develop a homemade blended formula for their child, they're honoring their role in deciding what foods will meet their child's nutritional needs. They learn how to create a nurturing environment for offering the formula, and discover the best times of day for giving the child a formula meal. As parents focus on expanding communication, they are able to understand what the child is saying about his or her interests, interactions and comfort level. This information enables fine-tuning of the what, where and when of mealtime responsibilities.

Learning to read and understand a child's nonverbal or verbal communication creates a partnership that enables the child to guide the meal. However, listening and understanding are not enough. We also must honor the child's communication.

When the child indicates a need for a pause in the meal, parents can respond by stopping the flow of food through the tube. The child might be taught to look at the tube or clamp as a signal to stop or start eating. One older child loved looking at stop-and-go signs that her father made for her. When she looked at the red stop sign, her mother stopped giving the food; when she looked at the green go sign, she received more food. Another child learned to recognize his own internal signals and delighted in having conversations with "Mr. Tummy." He would ask Mr. Tummy if he needed more food and tell his mother, "Mr. Tummy says stop" or "Mr. Tummy says go."

Children are responsible for how much they eat and whether they eat. Most tube fed children are dependent upon an adult to physically offer the formula in the same way that an infant is dependent upon a parent to offer food from the breast, bottle or spoon. Children who are fed orally say "no" and actively prevent food from entering their mouths. They clamp their mouths closed, push away the spoon and refuse to take any more. Children who are tube fed lack many of these options. The tube is already inserted into the stomach and the hole through which the food enters remains open, even when the child doesn't want to eat.

Tube fed children often discover other physical ways of saying "no." Gagging and retching may be the response of a child who is beginning to feel uncomfortable. The child may become physically tense and emotionally stressed from the fear of getting too much food or feeling sick. Children who increase tension in the abdomen, cry or develop irregular breathing patterns often find their tension will slow down or stop the flow of the formula. Their increased agitation during the meal can limit the amount of formula they receive, but it also increases gastrointestinal discomfort.

When children tell us that they want to stop eating, their parents often are fearful they won't eat enough to grow and be healthy. In addition, medical professionals typically tell parents that their child must have a specific number of ounces and calories at every meal. They state or imply that if parents don't give the full amount, the child will become ill or fail to thrive. This is a model used for giving medicine, not food. Many parents follow the medical prescription for food and continue to give the last ounce of formula, even if the child is on the verge of vomiting. Parents then become sad and frustrated because they have worked hard to get in the full eight ounces of formula and the child vomits the last four ounces. If they had listened to their child's signals to stop and ceased giving food after six ounces, more food actually may have been eaten.

All of the research literature and parent experience tells us that no child eats the same amount of food at each meal or each day. Over time children adjust their caloric and nutrient intake to meet their growth needs. They may eat a large amount at one meal and very little at the next since their intake is guided by internal appetite cues. Tube feedings typically offer the same amount of the same food at the same time each day. Many children are fed continuously at a very slow rate by a feeding pump. The lack of variation and the lack of child input into the meal contribute to a lack of hunger and satiation awareness in children. It can be helpful to offer different amounts and different foods during different tube feedings.

Children also may develop helpless and negative associations with mealtimes when their needs and communication aren't honored. When parents honor a child's emerging communication of comfort, discomfort, hunger and fullness, they support a more natural normal relationship with food and mealtimes.

Each child needs a basic number of calories and nutrients to support healthy growth. Parents need the reassurance that they're providing a diet that supports this growth. They can explore many creative ways to enable their child to receive enough calories in a 24-hour period without increasing stress levels during a specific meal.

Many parents say their children's gastrointestinal comfort increased when homemade blended formula was introduced. They had less retching, vomiting and mucous congestion. They had more normal bowel movements and accepted more food with little or no distress. Many had fewer illnesses, looked healthier and grew more rapidly than they had in the past.

Parents also report that it takes time to identify the best food combinations to include in the formula, the best scheduling and the best ways of offering the formula to their child. When they focus on developing a communication partnership with their children, this task becomes easier. Children lead the way and tell us what works and what doesn't. They're the best experts for their own bodies. When we listen and collaborate with them, our job becomes much easier and more efficient.

For additional information on communication signals see:

Klein, M.D. (2003). *The "Get Permission Approach to Mealtime and Oral-Motor Treatment*. VHS & DVD. Tucson, AZ: Mealtime Notions, LLC (www.mealtimenotions.com).

Morris, S.E. and Klein, M.D. (2000). Chapter 13–Learning and Communication at Mealtimes. *Pre-feeding Skills – A Comprehensive Resource for Mealtime Development 2nd ed.* Austin, TX: Pro-Ed.

For additional information on responsibility at mealtimes see:

Satter, E. (2000). *Child of Mine: Feeding with Love and Good Sense* (3rd ed.). Boulder, CO: Bull Publishing.

Satter, E. (1987). *How to Get Your Kid to Eat . . . But Not Too Much.* Boulder, CO: Bull Publishing.

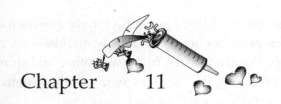

Mealtime Socialization and Homemade Blended Formulas

Chapter 11

Marsha Dunn Klein, M.Ed., OTR/L

Whether we eat by mouth or by tube, mealtimes are social times.

Mealtimes provide opportunities to dialogue with others, share thoughts and feelings, and to learn about mealtime routines and food preparation. Mealtimes are central to many celebrations and community get-togethers.

Children derive many benefits from sharing meals with different people in different situations. Active mealtime participation helps children who only get nutrition by tube to gain a broader understanding of food and its place in life while experiencing invaluable social interactions.

Mealtime Partners

Orally fed children eat with their parents, with brothers and sisters, as well as with relatives and friends. Often only one parent, the one who feels most comfortable with the tube and it's paraphernalia, feeds children who are fed by tube.

It's easy to miss out on the broader social picture of mealtime when mealtime partners are limited. Different people have different ways of offering food, different conversations and different emotions about mealtimes. Parents are encouraged to take turns in providing tube feedings so children have different partners for mealtime socialization.

Mealtime Preparation Routines

Children who are fed by tube often have limited experiences with food and mealtime preparation. Parents often don't involve tube fed children in the family routine of getting ready for a meal because they see tube feedings as very separate from family meals. But the tube fed child still can learn and benefit from engaging in mealtime routines. Although tube feeding typically doesn't offer a traditional place setting, serving

opportunity or clean-up process, tube fed children still can learn these routines. They can help set up, hold and clean up the tube feeding equipment. Some older children can even independently use syringes, extensions and pumps to feed themselves their formula, whether commercial or homemade.

Additionally, children who eat through tubes can participate, as they're able, with setting the family table by placing dishes at each place, or handing out straws or napkins. Some children can do this independently and others need considerable assistance. Many children serve themselves some of the family meal even if they aren't able or interested in actually eating any quantity. This helps them become familiar with smells, sights and textures of different foods, as well as sharing in the turn-taking of serving. Children can clean up after meals by clearing plates, or helping to put away the tube feeding materials.

Food Preparation

Children fed by tube experience food differently from oral eaters. Food often comes from a can or a blender. It's put directly into the stomach by a tube. They may never learn that there are individual foods with individual properties. By participating in the preparation of family foods, they can learn that the food in the tube is a blended version of real food; that an apple is red and hard and smells a lot like applesauce; that broccoli looks like little trees and is responsible for making their blended food mixture a green color; that cheese can be sliced or grated or cut into cookie cutter shapes and not just blended.

Children learn from handling food. They can help put spreads on bread or crackers, make and decorate cookies, stir flavored drinks and tear lettuce for a salad. They not only are learning to identify foods, but they're learning to become friendly with them. They learn the smell and texture well before checking out the taste.

Including children in the preparation of home-made blended formulas allows them to be part of their own nutritional routine. They can put food in the blender – smelling, touching and tasting it in the process! They can make beginning choices in the blend. "Do you want papaya or mango today?" "Would you prefer green beans or beets?"

Foods can be explored individually as they enter the blender. "Do you like the smell of peas or corn better?" "What color are these berries?" "Would you like a taste of this yogurt?" With these interactions children learn that mealtimes are not just about how many bites are eaten or tried. And mealtimes are not just about other people eating. Food preparation is a wonderful way to personalize food interaction.

Some families grow their own foods. Many tube fed children have enjoyed exploring in the garden. Digging in the dirt, helping to plant seeds, water and pick food can provide rich learning opportunities for any child, and especially those with limited food experiences.

Mealtime Modeling

Children learn much about eating from watching others. They see others using fingers and spoons, cups and straws, forks and chopsticks. They learn to use these utensils first by observation. They learn how different foods are eaten. Ice cream cones are for licking. Yogurt is for scooping. Chips are for dipping. Think about it. If children only have experience with formulas, how will they know what to do when interacting with a drumstick or a piece of corn on the cob? All children seem to be more willing to try these novel foods when they've seen others enjoy them.

Conversation and Sharing

Much of the socialization that occurs at meals lies in conversation and sharing. Talking about interesting subjects, activities of the day, things learned at school, upcoming family events and even news reports gives family members an opportunity to learn from each other and share while taking the focus away from "how many bites did you eat?" or "eat more food!"

Mealtime values, manners and turn taking are modeled and discussed. Children learn about their own families and what's important to them. Guidelines for what is or isn't acceptable at the family table are internalized. Children may discover through the example of a brother or sister that throwing food isn't allowed. Through this observation they learn that if they don't want any more formula, pulling out the tube and throwing it on the floor isn't acceptable; they may try other more socially acceptable ways of communicating that they're full and want to end the meal.

Celebrations

Most families have specific foods that traditionally are served at special family occasions such as birthdays, anniversaries and holidays. Children who are fed by tube can be actively involved with each of these social celebrations. Some parents choose to blend some cake and ice cream at a birthday party, some turkey and pumpkin pie at Thanksgiving, and some corned beef and cabbage on St. Patrick's Day. Family celebrations can provide opportunities for special mealtime alternatives that take the family out of the usual routine or recipe.

Families who have shared cultural and religious food preferences can include their tube fed children in these traditions. Most ethnic and religious groups have certain foods that are typically served at family or community meals. Pasta dishes often have Italian roots. Enchiladas and salsa bring to mind the food traditions of families from Mexico. Barbeque or country fried chicken conjure images of the southern United States. Variations of many of these foods are served at 4th of July picnics, church suppers, or special religious observances such as Shabbat, Christmas, or Ramadan. These foods can be modified and incorporated into a homemade blended formula. Potato pancakes and apple-sauce blend nicely for a Hanukkah meal. Hard-boiled or deviled eggs may be blended after an Easter egg hunt.

Community Meals

Children who are fed by tube can be included in the community aspects of food – the getting of food and the eating of food.

We obtain our food from many places in the community, such as grocery stores, bakeries and restaurants. Tube fed children can be included in the experience of seeing the choices and making decisions. "Shall we get some fresh pineapple or fresh strawberries?" " Shall we get this type of grain cereal?" "Look, these peas are dried, these come in a can and these are frozen." Bakeries and ice cream parlors are wonderlands of sights and smells. Choosing treats to bring home to share with siblings can be lots of fun. These foods can be touched or tasted along the way.

Restaurants can be sit-down events or fast food stops. Some families choose to complete tube feedings before going to a restaurant, providing primarily social conversation experiences while others are ordering food and eating. Others bring a blended or commercial formula to offer during the meal at a neighborhood cafe. Restaurants can also provide opportunities to offer different foods prepared by different people in a different setting. These foods can be handed to others, explored or tasted. Parents can create a "restaurant bag" that contains an assortment of dishes and utensils, books about eating and mouth toys for the child to explore during the meal.

Most families occasionally pick up a quick meal at a fast food restaurant. One family realized their three-year-old tube fed child was feeling left out of the fun of ordering at the drive-up window with her siblings. Her mother decided to let her daughter order her own cheeseburger, knowing full well that she didn't have the interest or skills to actually eat it. At first, Fionna would just hold

the wrapped burger, brimming with pride that she was doing the same thing that her siblings were doing. Over time, she would unwrap it, pick at it, smell it, lick it and gradually, as her oral skills improved, she would take little bites. As her homemade blended diet expanded, she eventually would participate in blending some of the burger with some milk and have it for lunch or dinner. Mother and daughter decided together that they would wrap up whatever Fionna didn't eat and put it in the freezer for her grandfather to eat when he came to visit. Whenever he arrived, Fionna would proudly share the piles of cheese-burgers that she and her mother had frozen! The point is that the social opportunity of ordering at the fast food restaurant was far more important to Fionna than the actual eating of the burger. She no longer was left out because she wasn't an oral eater. She was a proud part of the activity.

School is another community place where eating occurs. Children who eat by tube are often fed in the nurse's office. It's easy to whisk off a tube fed child to the nurse's office to provide calorie nourishment while other children are eating, but unfortunately the child then misses out on the social nourishment of mealtimes.

Some schools have the child participate in the snack or lunchtime with classmates, and then visit the nurse for a tube meal. Many nurses save some of their own lunch to eat at the same time, and the two engage in mealtime conversations. Some older children may desperately want to participate in the social aspects of the school cafeteria but cannot actually eat anything. They may bring a snack from home in their lunch boxes and lick the food or give tastes to friends. Others are given the tube feeding in the classroom or cafeteria with the other students. When this is done successfully, the child's parents have introduced the concept and talked about it with the child's classmates, giving them an opportunity to see, explore and understand how the familiar concept of eating can include taking food directly into their tummies.

Different Places and Spaces

Mealtimes look different and take on a different feel in different places. Eating at home is different than eating at a restaurant. Eating in the park on a blanket under a tree is different from eating at the zoo watching a family of monkeys. The environment feels different, smells different and the conversation is different.

It's easy to get in the habit of offering tube feedings in one particular corner of one particular room. By thinking about the bigger picture of mealtimes and their tremendous social value, parents may decide to diversify the place and the content of meals.

For additional information on tube feeding meals in the classroom see:

Klein, M.D. (2003) *Taking Tube Feedings to School.*
VHS & DVD. Tucson, AZ: Mealtime Notions, LLC.

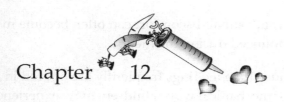

Chapter 12

Stress and Mealtimes

Suzanne Evans Morris, Ph.D, CCC

Many children and their parents experience high levels of stress in their lives. Physiological stressors such as surgery, illness, responses to medications, pain and lack of sleep influence the body's ability to function at an optimal level.

Emotional stress is derived from our perceptions and beliefs about the events and experiences that touch our lives. What's stressful for one person may not be stressful for another. It's possible to reduce stressful reactions by recognizing the situations and emotions that trigger them and consciously choosing a different perspective.

The Parent's Stress

Tube feedings offer a special set of potentially stressful situations for parents. Feeding tubes are typically recommended when infants or young children are simultaneously experiencing major medical challenges that limit their ability to swallow safely or to take in enough food and liquid to support adequate growth, nutrition and hydration. Parents frequently are mentally, emotionally and physically exhausted from their child's illness and the critical decisions that they have already made during this period. When the tube is recommended as part of the total medical solution during a period of hospitalization, the decision may be easier because it can be viewed as another medical solution that can save the child's life.

The meaning that parents attach to a feeding tube once the child is at home can be quite different and varied. The tube may be recommended when the child is not sick and is taking some foods orally. A mother may be spending hours at each meal trying to coax her child to eat more; and still the child does not gain enough weight. Feelings of guilt and a sense of personal failure may crop up when the doctor or dietitian recommends a

feeding tube. Many young women learned from parenting their baby dolls as toddlers that "a good mother can feed her child". This contributes to feelings of inadequacy and stress when her child is unable to eat enough to grow and thrive. Most parents are unfamiliar with the possibility that a child might be unable to eat by mouth. Before their baby was born they assumed their child would enjoy eating and have the skills and desire to eat a wide variety of foods. When they learn their child needs to eat through a feeding tube, they're faced with a profound sense of loss. Most people go through a grieving process as they face loss, whether the loss is of a relationship, a job, a death or a personal dream or assumption. The loss of eating and drinking is very powerful for many parents.

Tube feedings are accompanied by unfamiliar equipment and procedures. Learning to use feeding tubes, formulas, syringes, feeding bags and feeding pumps can initially feel overwhelming. This is particularly true if part of the system malfunctions or the child is uncomfortable during the meal.

Most parents understand when an orally fed child wants more food, needs a pause in the meal or has had enough to eat. There may be personal or cultural pressures to override the child's signals, but in most instances it is the child who makes the final decision. Reading the more subtle cues of an infant or toddler with a physical, sensory or gastrointestinal disability can be very challenging. As parents are trying to learn these cues and respect them, professionals may be telling them that their child must take in a specific number of calories at every meal. Their desire to regulate the timing and volume of the child's formula may be in conflict with their desire to follow the directions from the doctor or dietitian so their child will grow.

When children and adults don't feel well, their natural response is to eat less or to stop eating. Many children who have feeding tubes experience gastrointestinal discomfort. They may continue to retch and vomit even with tube feedings, and cry or fuss when food is offered by mouth or by tube.

Mealtimes can become highly stressful for parents who want to respect their child's signals of discomfort but feel that if they give less food, their child won't grow.

Many parents worry about the added costs that tube feedings create. Special formulas are extremely expensive when compared with breast milk, infant formulas or the meals typically served to toddlers and young children. Payment for feeding tubes, syringes, formula bags and pumps increases costs exponentially. Although many families are able to get help with these costs through private insurance, Medicaid or other third party payers, a substantial portion of the expenses still must be paid by the family. Insurance companies may limit the number of replacement feeding tubes that will be paid for each year or the number of syringes that will be supplied per month for bolus feedings. Many insurance companies will not pay for special formulas because they label them as food and not as a medical need. These financial pressures add to the stress that many families experience when their child has a feeding tube.

For all of these reasons, many parents want to wean their child from the tube as quickly as possible. They're drawn toward programs that promise rapid weaning or feel frustrated and angry when tube feedings appear to continue indefinitely.

The Child's Stress

Children may also feel stress at mealtimes. Often they have been given a feeding tube because they are ill or lack coordination and endurance for safe swallowing and growth. These situations may continue to influence their tube feeding mealtimes. Reflux, vomiting, retching and other

gastrointestinal discomfort can often become more pronounced during the meal.

Because tube feedings frequently are offered in a more mechanical way, children may experience the added discomfort of formula that comes in too quickly or continues to arrive when the stomach is filled.

Even though they may tell the person feeding them that they need to stop, they feel pressure from adults to eat more than is comfortable. Their communication signals may be ignored or misunderstood.

Individual Responses to Potentially Stressful Situations

Our society constantly reminds us that we're at the mercy of the people and events in our lives. We're taught verbally and by example that situations and people cause us to respond in predictable ways. But in fact the same situation can trigger different feelings and actions in different people.

A person's response to a specific situation is not a function of the event itself. Rather, the event stirs up a complex set of personal meanings and beliefs that are unique to each individual. Instead of responding to the event, each individual responds to these meanings and beliefs.

For example, the doctor has just recommended a gastrostomy tube for a child who is not growing well. Different parents respond in very different ways to this recommendation. One mother may feel very happy because she believes this will allow her child to grow. Or, she may feel relief because trying to get her child to eat enough by mouth has resulted in a constant battle and family conflict. Another parent may feel discouraged and upset because she believes she's a failure as a mother. Or she may be unhappy and angry with her child for refusing to eat by mouth. To her, accepting the tube feels like a defeat. She even may be angry about the tube because she's furious with the doctor, whom she believes never listens to her.

48

The same holds true for children. A child may experience uncomfortable physiological sensations from reflux and nausea and may respond to these sensations by falling asleep or by becoming upset, leading to gagging or retching. The child may become frightened and anticipate these distressing sensations, crying and tensing up even before the food is given.

Although we may have little control over the events in our lives, we always have the choice of how we will respond. We give a personal meaning to each event. We decide within ourselves whether the event is good or bad for us. When we choose a positive or optimistic meaning, we can approach the situation from a base of happiness. When we select the negative or pessimistic interpretation, we respond with unhappiness and increased stress. It all depends on what we believe – on the personal meaning that we give the experience.

Stress and Pain

Many children with gastrointestinal complications have chronic pain and discomfort during, after and between meals. When they have pain from gastroesophageal reflux, ulcers, poor digestion, abdominal dysfunction and stomach pressures associated with mealtimes, it's hard to want the food next time. We know from carefully watching children, as well as from research, that when pain or discomfort is associated with eating (by mouth or tube), appetite is suppressed.

Chronic pain creates a stress cycle that's detrimental to appetite, growth and any type of enjoyment at mealtimes. This occurs for several reasons. First, the pain itself diminishes a child's desire to eat. Second, when the process of eating increases discomfort, children learn to refuse food as a way of taking care of themselves. Instead of learning that eating is an enjoyable time, they learn the opposite – to move themselves away from eating! Third, pain shifts the way the body regulates itself. It creates an excitable "arousal" response in the body. The heart beats faster, blood pressure increases, and there is

disordered movement within the gastrointestinal system. This gastrointestinal disorder can include severe nausea, vomiting, slowed stomach emptying, no stomach emptying or too much movement in the intestines leading to cramping and diarrhea.

Typically a vicious cycle is activated – the pain leads to arousal, which leads to slow gastric emptying. The reduced gastric motility can lead to pain, which again can lead to arousal and the cycle continues.

Over time, it seems to take less and less pain or discomfort to create the same level of arousal in children. For many children just the fear and anticipation of the upcoming pain can cause a physical reaction of pain, even before the meal is presented.

Each child responds uniquely to the stimulus of pain, and the intensity that the child perceives is different for each individual. This perception is influenced by physical symptoms, the sensory perception of the symptoms, the arousal level through which the body responds to the pain and sensory perception, and the personal meaning that the child attaches to the pain.

For example, the child has recurrent inflammation in the esophagus and vomiting with eating (pain or discomfort). These symptoms can lead to disordered motility. The inflammation stimulates pain in the nerve that travels between the gastrointestinal tract and the spinal cord. The message then is passed to the nerve that travels up to the brain (sensory perception). The child perceives this sensation based on intensity, past experiences with this pain, parental reaction and the arousal response. Over time it takes less pain to elicit the same pattern of response. Pain, along with slowed motility, sensory perception, emotions and the child's responses are all interconnected, and very real for the child.

Treatment to improve comfort at mealtimes, therefore, will be influenced by multiple factors. Some professionals work primarily to change the diet, meal sizes and mealtime positions. Others use surgery and motility drugs to treat the way the gastrointestinal system physically works. Still others focus on reducing or eliminating the gastric acid that creates so many of the symptoms of inflammation and pain.

Many professionals help children develop skills in whole body relaxation, mental focus, breathing and distraction, to reduce the anticipation of pain and increase the child's control during the meal. Some physicians will focus directly on elimination of the pain response and anxiety through medications that help reduce the child's overall stress symptoms.

Stress and Growth

Mealtimes themselves often become the major trigger of stress reactions in children and parents. Foods which contribute to gastrointestinal discomfort or metabolic, allergic or hypersensitive reactions can create both physiological and emotional stress.

Fear can create a lower threshold for gagging and vomiting. When the child vomits food or formula, many parents become worried and frustrated. They're afraid their child won't receive enough calories and may even feel angry that they need to somehow get him to take more formula. Although the child's body has said "no more -- something's wrong," the parents' fears create pressure to take in more food. Children with feeding tubes are often verbally or nonverbally chastised for the amount they ingest orally or by tube. The message is frequently "it's not enough," which the child often interprets as "you're not good enough."

Children's bodies are programmed to take in nutrients and calories and use them for growth and health, but sometimes this program doesn't work well. Automatic growth of a child's body can be compared to a computer running software for growing. This growing program operates the body's ability to digest, breathe, eliminate and protect itself through the immune system.

But the body's computer also has a program for protection, and it switches from the growth program to the protection program whenever it feels threatened. Growing is no longer its highest priority when it perceives a situation as dangerous. Protecting itself becomes its main concern.

The body's protection system supports the ability to be strong enough to run away or stay and fight the attacker. In this "fight-or-flight" response the body directs its full energy and resources toward surviving. The body doesn't need to digest food and grow; it simply needs to survive. To do this, it must shut down the growth program temporarily. The brain does this by secreting a series of hormones that shift blood from the gastrointestinal system to the arms and legs. Digestion shuts down and stomach emptying is delayed. This increases the body's ability to get away from the dangerous situation or increase physical strength for fighting the danger.

The problem with this strategy is that it was designed for occasional situations of acute stress where real danger to survival is involved. This system is counter-productive when the body is under chronic stress. The body doesn't differentiate between acute and chronic stress. It simply gets a message from the brain advising it to prepare for danger. So a body designed to respond strongly when a tiger confronts it on the path now responds in the same way to situations that have nothing to do with immediate physical survival. We may have a fight-or-flight response when we don't have as much money as we want or when our children don't do their homework.

The bottom line is that chronic stress is directed by our perceptions and beliefs that a situation is dangerous or not in our best interest. The meaning we attach to the event determines our response, not the event itself. There are the added physiological and emotional stressors of environmental toxins, pharmaceutical drugs, poor nutrition, a busy lifestyle, work-related challenges, and the task of raising and caring for children with special needs. This means that stress hormones flood the body with messages that constantly tell it to protect itself.

In children, it also means there is less energy available for digesting and absorbing food and growing. This is highly relevant to the feeding and mealtime issues of children who receive tube feedings. A large percentage of these youngsters have challenges with the growth system. Respiratory, digestive, elimination and immune system problems are common. Many have measurable difficulty gaining weight and growing, despite receiving an appropriate number of calories.

Gastroesophageal reflux and other problems with the gastrointestinal system are common. Reflux contributes to nausea, vomiting and esophagitis. Infants and young children then associate this pain and discomfort with being fed, and learn to protect themselves by refusing to eat or limiting the amount of food they take in. Constipation occurs frequently, both as a result of inadequate fiber from a liquid formula diet and from an overall reduction in efficient function of the gastrointestinal system.

As part of the fight-or-flight response, specific hormones send a message to slow down digestion and stop stomach emptying. This contributes physiologically to the delayed gastric emptying that causes children to feel full all the time, because the stomach actually is full of the food from the last meal. A constantly full stomach also increases the likelihood of reflux and vomiting.

Stress at mealtimes interferes with digestion and growth. It also makes it more difficult for children to learn that mealtimes can be pleasurable and that food itself can be satisfying and nurturing.

Homemade Blended Formulas and Mealtime Stress

A homemade blended formula may reduce some of a child's physiological stress if the food itself contributes to a greater comfort level. Adults reduce some of their own stress when their child seems more comfortable and happier. They may feel more in control of their child's diet and enjoy making specific nutritious food choices.

Many families say the decision to give a homemade blended formula offers a feeling of relief that provides a major reduction in their stress level. However, the formula change needs to be placed into the broader environmental perspective of how the tube meal is given. This involves thinking about how to make the mealtime itself nourishing and nurturing for both the child and parent.

Creating a Nourishing Mealtime Environment

The environment in which the meal is offered can either increase or decrease stress levels for both the child and parent. When adults think about creating a good environment ahead of time, meals are easier for everyone because they're more positive and less stressful.

Attitudes and Intention

The attitude of the feeder plays a critical role in creating the overall atmosphere of the meal. When adults approach mealtime with the intention to be present, loving, nonjudgmental and happy they become more receptive to the child's communication signals and desire to become a partner.

Timing

Homemade blended formulas are usually given as bolus feedings with a syringe. Each child has specific needs for how much formula and the timing or speed with which the formula is offered. It's worth taking the time to find the most comfortable way of offering the meal.

Location

Sensory input and physical characteristics of the location selected for the meal play a major role in the child's comfort and physical control. If the environment matches the child's needs, tube feeding meals are more comfortable and successful.

Communication and Control

The only person who knows during the meal whether the homemade blended formula is creating comfort or discomfort is the child. All children are able to communicate what's happening inside their bodies through movements, signs or symbolic language.

It's up to the feeder to learn the child's special communication system and respond in a way that honors the child's messages. When children are able to have some control during a meal, their stress is reduced.

Tools that Support Stress Reduction

Tools that contribute to stress reduction can help both children and parents participate in a happier and more relaxed meal. Many of these tools are highly effective in reducing pain. Just as stress is triggered by different beliefs for different people, different tools may be effective for different adults and children.

Through asking some basic questions and observing the responses of both their child and themselves, adults often can find specific activities to incorporate at mealtimes, such as:

Music

Quiet, organizing music can help children and adults relax physically, mentally and emotionally. A specialized type of music called Metamusic® contains an auditory guidance system known as Hemi-Sync® that's based on binaural beats. Metamusic is particularly effective in reducing overall stress and helping children focus their attention in a positive way on what's going on in their bodies.

- What type of quiet, organizing music seems to relax the child?

- What type of quiet, organizing music supports the parent's relaxation and focus of attention?

Imagery

Imagery can create positive scenarios that both parents and older children can use to reduce stress. Research has shown that the brain is unable to tell the difference between an experience that occurs outside the body and one that occurs inside. Whether we look at a flower growing in our garden or imagine that same flower inside our heads, the brain responds with the same patterns of electrical activity.

Anytime we think of something in the future, we're using our imagination, simply because none of us ever know the future – even a future that is five minutes from now. People frequently imagine a future that they don't really want. They might create a make-believe scenario in their minds that includes their child being ill or refluxing and vomiting the meal.

It is possible, however, to imagine something desirable. Parents could go into a meal creating feelings and pictures in their heads of their child being happy and comfortable. They could imagine recognizing and responding to every communication cue their child offers.

- Could the parent become aware of negative images that are created before and during the child's meal? Can parents simply notice these thoughts and imagery without judging the thoughts or themselves?

- Could the parent consciously decide to imagine a positive mealtime experience? If unhappy thoughts and images arise, could the parent let them pass and focus on specific positive images of what is desired at the present moment?

- Does the child enjoy listening to stories? If so, could the parent make up stories during the meal that are positive and interesting to the child? Many of these stories could feature the child as a main character.

Breathing

When children and adults are feeling stress or discomfort, they often hold their breath and briefly stop breathing. They frequently tighten the muscles of their abdomen. This can increase their perception of pain and discomfort. Help children focus on their breathing and encourage them to keep their breathing movement easy and continuous. Then they're able to relax more easily and become calmer.

- What type of breathing pattern does the child use during the meal? Is there relaxed movement of the abdomen and the chest during breathing? Is there tension in the child's abdomen that comes and goes?

- Does the child hold his or her breath intermittently during the meal? Does this occur primarily with feelings of stress and anxiety?

- If the parent places a hand gently on the child's abdomen, is it easier to monitor breathing?

- Does the child respond with an easier, deeper or more continuous breathing pattern when the parent comments on the positive aspects of "keeping the breath moving"?

Caring for the Caregiver

Many parents believe that all of their personal resources, including time, money and health priorities should be invested in their child. They frequently don't prioritize time to care for their own needs. They may also believe that any time spent on nourishing themselves is selfish.

In reality, children and their parents are so interconnected that when a parent is stressed, tired and in poor health it affects the child, in the same way that a child's stress and health issues affect the parent.

What types of activity or non-activity does each parent find enjoyable and nourishing (i.e. reading, sleeping, walking, listening to music, taking bubble baths, spending time with spouse or friends)? Would the parent be willing to take some time each day or several days a week to enjoy a personal activity that replenishes personal energy and health? How could this be accomplished?

Sleep and Nutrition

Both children and their parents need sleep and strong nutritional support. Many children sleep poorly; when children don't sleep well, neither do their parents.

Busy parents often spend their waking hours tending to the needs of their children and feel that they don't have time to prepare nutritious meals for themselves and the rest of the family. The result is tired parents and children who lack the nutritional reserves to deal effectively with stress and prevent stressful situations.

Bedtime rituals and routines as well as sleep-promoting music played at bedtime and throughout the night are beneficial for many children. When children go to bed earlier, parents have more personal time for each other and for engaging in relaxing activities before they get into bed.

Homemade blended formulas can make a strong contribution to improved nutrition for the whole family. When parents work with a dietitian to create nutritious blended meals for their tube fed child, they often become more aware of ways in which homemade meals can be cooked for the whole family. Balanced meals created from healthy ingredients can be prepared in less than 30 minutes. They typically cost less than prepared foods purchased at the grocery store or restaurant.

Food supplements may be appropriate for some parents and children to build health at a cellular level of the body. The need and availability of good supplements can be discussed with your dietitian and health care providers. Healthy cells lead toward healthy tissues and organs and a higher level of wellness for the whole person. Stress weakens the immune system, often resulting in more frequent periods of illness for everyone in the family. Committing to a higher level of nutrition increases the body's resilience to stressful situations and can result in calmer meals.

- What resources are available to support the child's ability to go to bed at a reasonable hour, fall asleep easily and sleep throughout the night?

- What changes can the parents make in purchasing and preparing foods that are nutritious for everyone in the family?

- Would nutritional supplements be helpful in increasing the health and wellness of both the child and parents?

Reducing stress for both the child and parent increases the possibility of better health and growth. A homemade blended formula offered in a nourishing environment increases the probability that the child will experience less stress, will digest the formula more easily and will grow well.

For additional information on creating a nourishing environment see:

Klein, M.D. and Morris, S.E. (2007). Chapter 13 – Creating a Nourishing Environment for Tube Fed Meals. *Homemade Blended Formula Handbook*. Tucson, AZ: Mealtime Notions, LLC.

For additional information on the role of stress, digestion and growth see:

Hyman, P.E., Danda C.E. (2004). Understanding and Treating Childhood Bellyaches, *Pediatric Annals*, 33:2, p 97-104.

Justice, B. (1988). *Who Gets Sick: How Beliefs, Moods and Thoughts Affect Health*. Derbyshire: Peak Press.

Lipton, B.H. (2005). *The Biology of Belief: Unleashing the Power of Consciousness, Matter and Miracles*. Santa Rosa, CA: Mountain of Love/Elite Books

For additional information on our beliefs and attitudes see:

Kaufman, B. N. (1994) *Happiness is a Choice*, New York, NY: Ballantine Books.

Morris, S.E. (2007). The Happiness Option at Mealtimes. http://www.new-vis.com/fym/papers/p-feed22.http

For additional information on music and sound in stress reduction see:

Leeds, J. (2005). *The Power of Sound: How to Manage Your Personal Soundscape for a Vital, Healthy and Productive Life*. Rochester, VT: Healing Arts Press.

Morris, S.E. (1997). Opening the door with Metamusic®. In Schneck, D.J. and Schneck, J.K. ed. *Music in Human Adaptation*. Blacksburg, VA: Virginia Tech Press, p. 167 - 181. http://new-vis.com/fym/papers/p-lrn11.htm

For additional information on family meals and nutrition see:

Satter, E. (1999). *Secrets of Feeding a Healthy Family*. Madison, WI: Kelcy Press.

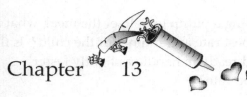

Chapter 13

Creating a Nourishing Environment For Tube Fed Meals

Suzanne Evans Morris, Ph.D, CCC

Physical and Emotional Nourishment

Many parents shift to a homemade blended formula because they believe the foods in the new formula will automatically improve their child's comfort and nutrition.

They may be drawn toward making their own formulas because they believe that a greater variation in food ingredients and the heavier weight of the homemade blended formula will increase their child's overall comfort during the meal. They perceive that a homemade meal can provide them with a wider variety of nutrients needed for growth.

Parents look primarily at physical nourishment that a blended formula can provide and see critically important elements and reasons for creating homemade blended formulas for their children.

But people experience nourishment at a much broader level. It can occur at the physical, mental, emotional and spiritual levels. Homemade blended formulas can be offered in the most nourishing environment possible for both youngster and parent.

What is nourishing for one person may not be nourishing for another. The specifics often depend upon past experiences and beliefs. A nourishing environment is not defined by specific equipment or elaborate procedures. The most universal aspects of a nourishing environment are attitudinal.

- We feel nourished when others are fully present and listening to what we're communicating.

- We feel nourished when another person unconditionally loves us.

- We feel nourished when our choices are respected.

- We feel nourished when we're accepted for who we are and are not judged by others.

- We feel nourished when we feel that we have some control over our own lives.

Homemade blended formulas contribute to the emotional nourishment of both parents and their children. Many parents speak of preparing the child's meal with love and a sense of empowerment in being able to make critical decisions about creating their child's formula. They're able to include their child in making homemade meals in a way that supports a sense of emotional connection for both parent and child.

Creating a Nourishing Mealtime Environment

Before offering a tube fed meal to a child, consciously think about the many ways to create an environment that provides physical, emotional and mental nourishment. When the environment provides nourishment rather than stress, children are able to learn more easily and grow and thrive.

Attitudes and Intention

Parents can set an intention to have a happy meal with their child, letting go of worries and unhappy thoughts for the short mealtime they share. They simply can choose to be present and not thinking about other things during this time with their child. They can decide to accept whatever happens during this specific meal, and see the child in a loving, non-judgmental way. By holding this intent and giving it top priority, adults are more able to be receptive to children's communication signals and respond as the child's mealtime partner.

Location

Choosing a supportive location for the meals is important. Consider and select choices that fit the child, parents and family.

- Will the child share a quiet meal with one parent, or while sitting at the table with the entire family?

- Does the child become overly excitable or over-loaded if the environment is noisy or very busy, or does he need a more visually active environment to stay interested and focused on the meal?

- Is the child more comfortable when the tube feeding is given lying down or sitting up?

- Can the child be helped to focus primarily on sensations of stomach comfort, discomfort, hunger or fullness. Is the child ready for small amounts of food by mouth while the stomach fills with formula?

The answers to these and many other location questions depend solely on the child and family situation. To find answers and solutions that provide the greatest comfort and support, look for answers that meet the greatest number of needs for everyone, not just the child.

Timing

In most cases homemade blended formulas are given as bolus feedings with a syringe. Meals may be offered to some children through pump feedings if the formula is relatively thin and the length of the meal is two hours or less.

There are many questions and choices to explore to find the most comfortable way of offering the meal.

- Does the child prefer to be offered very small amounts of formula evenly over a specific period of time, or offered slightly larger amounts with pauses in between?

- Does varying the amount of food given in a bolus support the child's comfort, or is comfort greater if the size of a bolus and length of pauses are regular?

- If using a pump to deliver the meal, what is the best rate and timing for the child? Is the child ready to handle a slightly faster pump rate?

Communication and Control

It's essential to choose a supportive way of encouraging communication and to offer a partnership that provides real choices during the meal. Many parents and professionals already have developed their ability to recognize and understand a child's verbal and non-verbal signals at mealtimes. Others are just beginning to consider the possibility that the child really has something to say. Research suggests that adults and children experience more stress when they perceive they have little control over an aspect of their lives. Less control also is associated with higher levels of illness, depression and learned helplessness. Because tube feedings are typically offered with adults providing all of the control and decision-making, children may feel added stress. Even when parents read their signals of comfort or discomfort, many children do not experience that these signals are honored.

As parents and professionals, we can begin to gently question our own beliefs about listening to children and following their lead while still providing them with safe limits.

- Are we able to recognize the child's earliest signals for discomfort or fullness, or must the child become severely uncomfortable or distressed before we notice there's a problem?

- Are we willing to listen to the child and stop the flow of formula at the first indications of discomfort or fullness?

- Is the child ready to help prepare the formula meal and choose specific foods to add to the formula?

- What are the easiest, most meaningful ways to help children know they're valued partners at the meal?

Stress Reduction

Stress influences both the physical and emotional nurturance of children.

When parents feel stress around mealtimes, they communicate this to their children. Young children and those who are nonverbal are especially astute at picking up the nonverbal messages communicated through the stress of their parents.

Stress contributes to poor gastrointestinal function. Food can stay in the stomach for long periods due to delayed gastric emptying. The movements of the stomach and intestines that are essential for easy and rapid passage of food may be diminished or halted for varying periods because stress causes the body to shift from a growth mode into a protection mode. Food may be poorly digested and assimilated, resulting in poor physical growth despite receiving appropriate calories and nutrients in the diet.

Reducing stress at mealtimes for both the child and parent increases the possibility of better health and growth. When a homemade blended formula is offered in a nourishing environment, it increases the probability that the child will feel better and will adapt well to the new diet.

For additional information on creating a nourishing environment see:

Klein, M.D. and Morris, S.E. (2007). Chapter 12 – Stress and Mealtimes. *Homemade Blended Formula Handbook*. Tucson, AZ: Mealtime Notions, LLC.

Morris, S.E. and Klein, M.D. (2000) Chapter 13–Learning and Communication at Mealtimes. *Pre-Feeding Skills – A Comprehensive Resource for Mealtime Development 2nd Ed*. Austin, TX: Pro-Ed.

For additional information on our beliefs and attitudes see:

Kaufman, B. N. (1994). *Happiness is a Choice*, New York, NY: Ballantine Books.

Justice, B. (1988). *Who Gets Sick: How Beliefs, Moods and Thoughts Affect Health*. Derbyshire, UK: Peak Press.

Morris, S.E. (2007). *The Happiness Option at Mealtimes*. http://www.new-vis.com/fym/papers/p-feed22.htm

Chapter 14

A Parent's Perspective: Family Involvement In Homemade Blended Formulas

Tina Valente

Joey was born in December 1996, right after Christmas. He is an only child who lives at home with both of his parents and a little black kitten with green eyes named Shego.

Joey loves to play outside. We have a pool in our back yard and swimming is his favorite summertime activity. He likes to ride his bike, play baseball and basketball with his dad, and hike in the desert. Joey just started taking karate lessons. He's practicing his moves and wants to earn a black belt someday. Joey loves to play his Gameboy®, eat popcorn, collect rocks, play miniature golf and bowl, and play on the computer. He works hard in school and on his homework. He is an excellent reader and speller, and likes math. He is kind and caring and worries when someone else is hurt or upset. He makes friends easily and is very outgoing. He loves to tell knock-knock jokes and to laugh.

We are a very "typical" family that just happens to have a child who receives his nutrition by tube. It's important to me to describe my son and some of his many wonderful qualities before talking about his feeding tube. Tube feeding will most likely be a lifelong reality for Joey. We do not, however, define our child or our lives solely by his medical condition or feeding tube. We have come to believe that it's important to strike a balance in our lives between the reality of Joey's medical needs and our family mealtime experiences.

Joey was born with a genetic liver disease called Alagille's syndrome. In addition, he has a number of gastrointestinal issues that complicate his life including severe gastroesophageal reflux, slow stomach emptying and malabsorption of fats and vitamins. Eating has been difficult from birth and Joey was soon classified as "failure to thrive." At 7 months he received a nasogastric tube for supplemental feedings and a more permanent gastrostomy tube at 9 months.

Joey has had continual feeding therapy over the years to promote his oral skills and improve his relationship with food. Unfortunately, it became obvious to all of us after a few years that it was unlikely that Joey would grow out of his reflux and the circumstances that caused it, as we had hoped. Though he does eat some foods orally, he has very little appetite and often does not feel well enough to eat. The majority of his nutrition, therefore, continues to be supplied by his tube.

Joey receives five to six supplemental bolus feedings daily to provide the calories and nutrition he needs. Our goal has been to make his bolus feeding less like a medical procedure and to involve him in the social and emotional aspects of family mealtimes.

For Joey, eating orally is a constant challenge. When he's feeling well, he's physically capable of eating almost any type of food that interests him. When he isn't feeling well, which is quite often, food is of no interest to him. Foods often taste differently to him due to his liver disease and many foods that most kids love, Joey finds very unappetizing. He also has had a great deal of sensory sensitivity since he was born and many textures of foods bother him or cause him to gag. We often feel like we're making progress with Joey's oral eating, only to feel defeated a few weeks later when he will get sick and avoid food for days or weeks at a time.

Regardless of how Joey is feeling about food, we make an effort to involve him in family mealtime. Even if he has no desire to eat, he still can be involved in the family activities that revolve around food. He enjoys emptying the dishwasher and setting the table. He also loves to stand on his little stool at the kitchen counter and help with preparing a meal. He particularly loves baking cookies, even though he typically doesn't eat them. We bake many batches of cookies to give as gifts.

When we sit down as a family for a meal, Joey doesn't always want to eat, however he still can participate in family time and conversation. Holiday meals are especially exciting for him. We set the dining room table with all the fancy dishes, candles and sometimes even wine glasses. We put a little soda in Joey's wine glass and he feels important and involved just like any other child would. He may only take a sip from his glass, or a few tastes from his plate, but he is truly engaged in the family experience of the holiday meal.

We also make an effort to give him a sense of control regarding food whenever possible. He enjoys shopping at the grocery store and I will ask him questions regarding the meal planning. "What should we make for dinner tonight? Chicken or pork chops?" He also enjoys the finger foods and samples that are often offered at the store. It's a great chance for an introduction to a food he may never have tried before. He may be only interested in smelling the sample or licking it, however there's something about having it offered to him at the store that makes it more appealing than having it offered at home.

Joey also enjoys the occasional fast food meal like every other child. The toy that accompanies the meal is the main attraction, however he typically will try a few bites of the meal before receiving the toy. We usually make a deal beforehand to share the meal, alleviating my frustration regarding wasting food if he doesn't eat much of the meal.

School is another great place to give Joey some control over his relationship with food. He attends a public school and currently is in third grade. Food is a very social part of a typical school day. Every morning I pack a sack lunch as well as a snack for him to eat orally. I give him choices regarding what I pack. "Do you want apple slices or carrots?" "Do you want butter-scotch pudding or a fruit roll up?" He "eats" his snack and his lunch with his classmates. Often most of the food comes back home in his lunch bag. However, watching his peers eat certainly influences and motivates him to eat some of what I have packed.

This year he has even started asking to have the school lunch when they're serving something that all the kids like. "Pizza Day" is a particular favorite. He may only eat a few bites, however we view this as a positive food experience that helps foster a better relationship with food.

Once Joey has had the opportunity to eat with his peers, he heads to the nurse's office to receive a supplemental bolus feeding through his tube. Twice a day, after snack and after lunch, the school nurse bolus feeds him. He typically carries an unfinished portion of his snack or lunch with him and will continue nibbling while in the nurse's office. Often, the nurse also eats part of her snack or lunch while Joey is in her office, to help provide a sense of a mealtime around the bolus feeding.

At home, we live by a "taste it" rule. We request that Joey "tastes" whatever is offered to him on his plate. A taste may be as little as a lick or as much as a bite. On occasion if a food is particularly challenging for him, "taste it," means smell it a few times. This rule occasionally leads to a love for some new food that was previously perceived as "yucky." After having the opportunity to eat orally, he receives his bolus meal. Typically this meal takes place at the family dinner table or wherever the family is eating, including eating out.

There are occasions where the "taste it" rule and the idyllic family meal scenario falls apart. We've learned that flexibility is a key ingredient in involving a tube fed child in family meals. At times, Joey's reflux is so acute that it's difficult for him to even sit at the table. Just the smell of foods will make him gag at these times. Bolus feeding also can be difficult at times when he's not feeling well. Often, a distraction such as watching a video while being fed helps these meals run more smoothly. We've decided that this is okay for our family. Joey doesn't sit with us for every single meal, however we do have family traditions and routines involving food in which our son can participate.

During a time in Joey's life when oral eating was particularly challenging, we turned our attention to the idea of improving his and our relationship with foods by using a homemade formula as an option for supplemental bolus feedings. We now include many different table foods in his formula. Often what he doesn't finish at the table is blended up and used in his tube. Joey receives a wide variety of foods that would be *extremely* difficult to get a typical nine year old to eat, such as salmon, avocado, flax seed, broccoli, cabbage and kale.

There has been a huge emotional benefit to the whole family connected to our homemade formula choice. The sense of frustration that I once felt about "left-over food " is gone. I also have a new sense of control and pride in knowing that I'm providing Joey with the very best nutrition possible. It's another opportunity for him to have some control over food choices. We involve him in the preparation of the homemade formula and it's empowering for him to help decide what goes into the blender and eventually his stomach. For example, he can decide if he wants peaches or pears or carrots or green beans. He also enjoys blending up food that's left on his plate. He has the satisfaction of feeling that he finished his meal like everyone else.

Today Joey is a happy outgoing nine year old. His social relationship with food continues to grow and expand. He's able to attend birthday parties and other social activities with his peers where food is an important factor. He typically will try what's offered to him and, on most occasions, others around him don't realize that he's a tube fed child. He will most likely need his gastrostomy tube for supplemental feedings for the rest of his life, however he can continue to learn to enjoy food in a social context since our world is one where food is central to many social events.

We have made peace with the fact that our family sometimes does things a little differently at mealtimes. We have developed mealtime routines that work for us and that help keep us connected as a family.

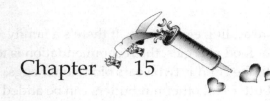

Chapter 15

Food Guidelines

Jude Trautlein, R.D. and Ellen Duperret, R.D.

This chapter will discuss basic food and nutrition guidelines for children. An understanding of food and nutrition is important when considering a move towards a homemade blended formula diet.

This is general information. Each child has unique nutritional needs, so it's important to work with a registered dietitian (R.D.) to ensure that individual requirements are met. The child's weight, age, physical activity, health status and special dietary requirements influence daily nutritional needs.

Nutrition can be broken down into macronutrients (proteins, fats, carbohydrates and water), micro-nutrients (vitamins and minerals), fiber and energy.

Proteins

Dietary protein provides amino acids: the building blocks for muscle, bone, cartilage, blood and other body fluids, enzymes and hormones.

Amino acids can be classified into essential (ones that cannot be produced by the body and must come from the diet) and nonessential (ones that can be made by the body). Protein sources, which provide essential amino acids, are important parts of a homemade blended formula.

In general, animal proteins such as cooked eggs, milk, meat, chicken and fish supply essential amino acids. (Uncooked eggs are not safe to use in homemade blended formulas because of the risk of illness from salmonella.)

Vegetable proteins from nuts, beans, and grains are an important part of a healthy diet. However, they don't individually supply adequate amounts of all essential amino acids. If a family chooses to provide a vegetarian diet for their tube fed child, particularly if a vegan diet is given, it's essential to have a solid knowledge of balancing a diet with vegetarian foods that provide the proper balance of amino acids.

How Much Protein Do Children Need?

Protein needs are determined by a child's age, weight and gender.

Daily Recommendations for Protein

Infant 7-12 mos.	1.5 gms protein/kgram*/day
Children 1-2 yrs.	1.1 gms protein/kgram*/day
Children 3-8 yrs.	.95 gms protein/kgram*/day
Males 9-13 yrs.	.95 gms protein/kgram*/day
Males 14-18 yrs.	.85 gms protein/kgram*/day
Females 9-13 yrs.	.95 gms protein/kgram*/day
Females 14-18 yrs.	.85 gms protein/kgram*/day

*Kilograms can be calculated by taking the weight in pounds, divided by 2.2.
Source: Food and Nutrition Board,
The National Academies of Sciences

For example, a 9-year-old boy weighing 60 pounds would have the following protein needs:
60 pounds divided by 2.2 = 27 kilograms
27 kilograms times 0.95 = 25 gms protein/day

How Much Protein Do Foods Contain?

Here are some examples of the protein content of common foods used in blended diets.
(See also, Appendix C - Food Sources of Proteins)

1 oz. beef, pork, poultry or seafood = 7–9 grams

1 egg = 6 grams

1 oz. cheese = 6 grams

½ cup cottage or ricotta cheese = 13-14 grams

1 cup yogurt = 7-13 grams

1 cup milk (skim, 1%, 2% or whole) = 8 grams

1 tbsp. peanut butter = 4 grams

½ cup tofu = 2-3 grams

½ cup cereal, pasta, or potato = 1-3 grams

½ cup rice = 2-3 grams

½ cup beans = 6-11 grams

1 slice bread or 1 tortilla = 2-3 grams

½ bagel = 4.5 grams

½ cup cooked or 1 cup raw vegetables = 2-4 gms

Meat and Beans Group

Foods from the meat and beans group supply protein, iron, B vitamins, and trace minerals. To prepare poultry, fish and meat for a homemade blended formula, trim excess fat and skin, cook thoroughly and puree with some broth. Dried beans are a good source of fiber and must be cooked until soft before pureeing. Tofu (soybean curd) is an easy addition to homemade blended formulas. Cooked egg yolks can be added after the child is nine to ten months of age, however it's advisable to wait until a child is at least 12 months old before adding egg whites. If there's a family history of food allergies, the recommendation is to wait until the child is two years old to offer eggs. Peanut butter and other nut butters can be added after a child is one year old, if there is no family history of food allergy. Otherwise, the recommendation is to wait until the child is three years old to offer them.

Milk and Milk Substitutes

Milk and milk products supply protein, calcium, phosphorus, riboflavin, niacin, Vitamin A, and when milk is fortified, Vitamin D. Children under one year of age may be offered breast milk or infant formula; other milks are not advised. After one year of age (or a year corrected age if the child was premature), cow's milk and other dairy products can be introduced.

Milk/ Milk Substitutes	Amount	Calories	Protein	Fat	Carbo	Calcium
Whole milk	1 cup	150	8 g	8 g	11 g	276 mg
2% milk	1 cup	120	8 g	5 g	11 g	285 mg
1% milk	1 cup	100	8 g	3 g	11 g	290 mg
Skim milk	1 cup	85	8 g	0 g	11 g	302 mg
Evaporated whole milk	1 cup	300-400	17-18 g	10 g	13 g	329 mg
Soy milk	1 cup	80-120	7 g	3 g	8 g	368 mg
Rice milk	1 cup	120	1 g	3 g	22 g	300 mg
Goat's milk	1 cup	168	9 g	10 g	11 g	326 mg
Almond milk	1 cup	70	2 g	3 g	1 g	240 mg
Coconut milk, canned	1 cup	445	5 g	48 g	6 g	41 mg
Nonfat dry milk, prepared	1 cup	81	8 g	0 g	11.8 g	279 mg
Nonfat dry milk, powder	1 Tbsp	16-27	1.5-2.5 g	0 g	2-4 g	53-95 mg
Yogurt, plain from whole milk	1 cup	140-180	7-13 g	7.4 g	11 g	300 mg

Resources: Nutritionist Pro™ Nutrition Analysis Software from Axxya Systems www.nutritionistpro.com (used with permission), and USDA Dietary Guidelines for Americans 2005 at www.health.gov/dietaryguidelines/

Children with lactose intolerance may be able to consume yogurt (which is lower in lactose than milk), lactose-reduced or lactose-free milk. For the child with a cow's milk allergy, fortified rice or soymilk or soy-based formula may be substituted. If a child also has a soy allergy, a hypoallergenic formula can be used.

Fats

Fats are an important part of the diet because they supply essential fatty acids ("essential" meaning that the body cannot make them). Twenty-five to 40% of the energy in a child's diet should come from fats. Children under three years of age have a greater need for fat because it's necessary for brain development. Fats are a source of concentrated energy, supplying nine calories per gram, as opposed to four calories per gram from proteins and carbohydrates. They help with the transport and absorption of fat-soluble vitamins (A, D, E and K), and provide satiety after a meal.

Fats stay in the stomach longer than proteins and carbohydrates, decreasing hunger between meals. Since they tend to slow stomach emptying, diets high in fat can aggravate symptoms of gastroesophageal reflux disease (GERD).

There are three classifications of fats: monounsaturated, polyunsaturated (including omega-3 and omega-6 fatty acids), and saturated (including trans fats). From a nutritional standpoint, monounsaturated fats and omega-3 fatty acids are the most healthful.

Monounsaturated fats provide essential fatty acids and are associated with a reduced risk of some cancers and cardiovascular disease. The best sources include olive oil, canola oil, avocado, most nuts and nut butters.

Polyunsaturated fats also provide essential fatty acids, in particular omega-6 and omega-3. Prefer-ably, the diet should contain a 3:1 ratio (or less) of omega-6 to omega-3. Western diets tends to con-tain an unhealthy balance of omega-6 to omega-3 (10-20:1). This imbalance of omega-6 to omega-3

can cause a lowering of both good cholesterol (HDL) and bad cholesterol (LDL). A diet higher in omega-3 fatty acids may improve cardiovascular health and reduce inflammatory processes.

Foods containing omega-3 fatty acids include flax, hemp oil, canola oil, pumpkin seeds, walnuts, and oily cold-water fish* such as salmon, tuna, cod and mackerel. Flax can be in the form of flax seeds, flax meal (ground flax), or flaxseed oil. Flax can easily be added to homemade blended formula. Make sure to store it in the refrigerator.

Common Monounsaturated Fat Food Sources

> Extra virgin olive oil
> Canola oil
> Most nuts and nut butters
> Avocado

Common Omega-3 Food Sources

> Flax (seed, meal, oil)
> Canola oil
> Pumpkin seeds
> Walnuts
> Cold-water fish such as salmon, tuna,
>   cod, mackerel*
> Hemp oil

*Fish contains some mercury, and should be eaten in moderation. Salmon can be eaten three to four times weekly, tuna and cod two to three times weekly, and mackerel once a month.
(See also, Appendix D - Food Sources of Fats)

Ideally, saturated fats are used only in minimal amounts because they've been shown to contribute to cardiovascular disease and some cancers. They're found in animal sources including butter, lard, meat, poultry skin, cheese, cream and whole milk.

Saturated fats also come from plants like coconut and palm oils. Many families believe that coconut oil has beneficial health properties because of the claims made by sellers. But these claims haven't met the standards for recommendation by the FDA (Food and Drug Administration) and the American Heart and Academy of Nutrition and Dietetics do not endorse its use as of this writing.

Trans fats are a type of saturated fat that is made by hydrogenating or partially hydrogenating vegetable oils. Margarines and many processed foods may contain trans fats. Saturated fats raise the LDL cholesterol and lower the HDL cholesterol, so moderation is recommended. Check labels to avoid purchasing foods that contain trans fats, hydrogenated fats or partially hydrogenated fats.

Carbohydrates

Carbohydrates are important in the diet as an energy source. Adequate carbohydrate intake ensures that dietary protein will be available for its essential functions. About half of the calories in a healthy diet come from carbohydrates. Carbohydrates can be classified as simple or complex. Simple carbohydrates (sugars) are broken down rapidly and provide quick energy. Complex carbohydrates (starches) provide more lasting energy and need to be a large part of a child's diet.

Examples of foods high in simple carbohydrates are candy, fruit, soda, juice and milk. With the exception of fruits and milk, sugars are mostly empty calories, which means that they provide energy but don't add much nutritional value. Too many sugars in the diet can promote obesity. Careful use of sugars is advised in homemade blended formula.

Examples of complex carbohydrates are breads, cereals and grains, pasta, tortillas and crackers. The whole grain varieties have more micronutrients and fiber, and help reduce constipation.

Grains

Whole grains and enriched refined grains are important sources of B vitamins and iron. Grains include wheat, oats, rice, barley, millet, couscous, bulgur, rye and quinoa. Whole grains contain the entire grain kernel (the bran, the germ and the endosperm). Examples are 100 percent whole wheat flour, steel cut oats, cracked wheat (bulgur), whole grain cornmeal and brown rice.

Refined grains are milled, which removes the bran and the germ. White rice, all-purpose flour and white bread are examples of refined grains. Refining gives the grain a longer shelf life and finer texture, but it also removes dietary fiber, some of the B vitamins and iron. Many of these refined grains are enriched, meaning thiamin, niacin, iron, riboflavin and folic acid are added back in after refining.

Grains will go through a feeding tube if the food is cooked thoroughly and blended; slow cookers work well for this.

Vegetables and Fruits

Vegetables and fruits are good sources of vitamins A and C, iron, trace minerals, fiber and phytonutrients. Fruits and vegetables can be fresh, frozen, canned or dried. Steaming is preferred to preserve vitamins when cooking vegetables.

Many orally fed children don't eat enough fruits and vegetables. Tube fed children can have a very healthy diet when fruits and vegetables are included in their homemade blended formulas.

Water

More than half the body is composed of water and getting adequate amounts is very important for tube fed children. Water helps the body filter out and eliminate waste products, and lubricates the joints. Getting adequate water helps decrease constipation.

Inadequate water intake can cause tiredness, headaches, dizziness, weakness and decreased immune response. Urine becomes very concentrated (dark yellow and strong smelling) when fluid intake is insufficient. The pediatrician and dietitian can help families to determine how much water a tube fed child needs.

Vitamins, Minerals and Phytonutrients

Micronutrients are substances that the body needs in very small amounts in order to grow and stay healthy. They include water-soluble and fat-soluble vitamins, minerals and phytonutrients. For a specific list of vitamin and mineral needs for different ages, see Appendix F – Vitamin Chart and Appendix K – Mineral Chart.

The terms "phytonutrient" and "phytochemical" currently are being used interchangeably to describe those plant compounds thought to have health-protecting qualities. This is an exciting area of research. The antioxidant, immune-boosting and other health-promoting properties of active compounds in plants are being investigated. A diet plentiful in a variety of brightly colored fruits and vegetables will provide a range of phytonutrients for good health.

Fiber

Fiber is the indigestible part of plants. It's a valuable component of a homemade blended formula because it improves intestinal health and aids in elimination. Good sources of fiber include cooked dried beans, whole grains, fruits and vegetables. (See Appendix E - Food Sources of Dietary Fiber.)

Recommended Dietary Allowance for Fiber for Children	
Age	Dietary Fiber
1-3 years	19 grams per day
4-8 years	25 grams per day
9-13 years, males	31 grams per day
14-18 years, males	38 grams per day
9-13 years, females	26 grams per day
14-18 years females	26 grams per day

*Based on 2002, the Food and Nutrition Board of the National Academy of Sciences Research Council issued Dietary Reference Intakes (DRI) for fiber

Calories/Energy

How do parents know if their tube fed child is getting enough calories? How would parents know if their orally fed child were getting enough calories? They would watch the child's overall energy level and monitor growth with the pediatrician. Growth can be evaluated by following the child's weight, height and head circumference on a growth chart. There are standard National Center for Health Statistics (NCHS) growth charts as well as specialty growth charts for children born prematurely, and those with Down syndrome and other medical conditions. A doctor or dietitian can recommend the appropriate growth chart for each child.

Calories are the energy provided in proteins, carbohydrates and fats. Proteins and carbohydrates contain four calories per gram, and fats contain nine calories per gram. Sufficient calories are needed for growth and to prevent the body from drawing energy from the protein in muscles (protein sparing).

When designing homemade blended formulas, it's valuable for families to work with a dietitian to set an appropriate calorie goal. This is an estimate based on the child's age, gender, weight, activity level, growth and medical histories. It's only an estimate, a starting point. When the growth chart shows a consistent upward curve, then the child is receiving adequate calories. If a child's weight gain has been too slow, then additional energy will be needed to improve the growth pattern.

Increased energy intake may be achieved by:

- Increasing the calories per ounce of formula. This often is done by adding fat, which increases energy without a large increase in volume.
- Increasing the volume of formula or number of boluses per day.

It's important to observe the child's tolerance of increased calories. If the child gags, retches, vomits, feels discomfort, or has undesirable bowel changes, then it's necessary to step back and proceed more slowly.

ChooseMyPlate

ChooseMyPlate is a graphic representation of a healthy diet. The Website ww.choosemyplate.gov© allows parents to input individual information about their child, and then provides a personalized plan that lists the recommended servings from each food group. The ChooseMyPlate plan suggests daily and weekly dietary food recommendations based on age, calories and level of activity.

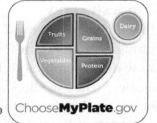

Dietary Supplements

Dietary supplements include standard multivitamins, teas, herbs and other formulations. Children's chewable multivitamin and mineral supplements can be crushed and added to homemade blended formula.

Some healthcare professionals are skeptical of the benefits of supplements, while others embrace their use. If the child is using ANY supplements, it's important to inform the physicians and registered dietitian. It's possible to overdose on vitamins. Some supplements can interfere with the absorption of medications and nutrients. Other supplements may have adverse effects and need to be stopped two weeks prior to surgery.

Ideally, children will receive all the nutrients they need from food. Food is the best source of nutrition, as other compounds in food are believed to aid in the absorption and utilization of nutrients. But in some cases, it's difficult or impossible for children to meet their needs solely through food and supplementation is needed. This is a decision that can be made with the help of the child's healthcare team.

For additional information on specific nutrition guidelines see:

Klein, M.D. and Morris, S.E. (2007). Chapter 16 – Homemade Blended Formulas and Hydration. *Homemade Blended Formula Handbook.* Tucson, AZ: Mealtime Notions, LLC.

Klein, M.D. and Morris, S.E. (2007). Chapter 31 – Vegetarian Children. *Homemade Blended Formula Handbook.* Tucson, AZ: Mealtime Notions, LLC.

Morris, S.E. and Klein, M.D. (2000) Chapter 16–Issues of nutrition. *Pre-feeding Skills – A Comprehensive Resource for Mealtime Development 2nd ed.* Austin, TX: Pro-Ed.

United States Department of Agriculture. (2010). Dietary Guidelines for Americans. (www.health.gov/dietaryguidelines). (www.choosemyplate.gov).

For additional information on applying the concept of ChooseMyPlate to the development of individual homemade blended formulas see:

Klein, M.D. and Morris, S.E. (2007). Chapter 25 – Anatomy of a Recipe. *Homemade Blended Formula Handbook.* Tucson, AZ: Mealtime Notions, LLC.

Klein, M.D. and Morris, S.E. (2007). Chapter 26 – Core Guidelines for a Homemade Blended Formula. *Homemade Blended Formula Handbook.* Tucson, AZ: Mealtime Notions, LLC.

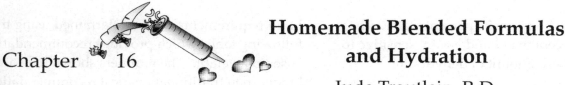

Chapter 16

Homemade Blended Formulas and Hydration

Jude Trautlein, R.D.

Everyone needs fluids for optimal health. When considering a homemade blended formula, the child's hydration needs should be carefully considered and monitored.

Water is important for many body functions, including temperature regulation and bowel movements. It's the major component of blood, digestive juices, urine, perspiration and mucus. It's contained in lean muscle, fat and bones.

The body needs water to maintain the health of every cell. Water helps eliminate the byproducts of metabolism and waste, keeps mucus in the lungs and mouth moist, lubricates joints, helps digestion, moisturizes the skin and carries nutrients and oxygen to the cells.

The body takes in water from foods such as fruits and vegetables, as well as from liquids. Fluids such as milk, juice or commercial formula support hydration needs, as do foods that are liquid at room temperature such as Jell-O, ice cream and soups. Using a combination of other fluids AND additional water seems to work best for most families.

While all children need fluids, some may need more than others. More fluids are needed when children have a fever, chronic diarrhea, vomiting or excessive drooling. Children require more fluids in hot weather or in warm, dry climates. Increased sweating—due to the weather, strenuous exercise or increased muscle activity such as spasticity—increases fluid needs. High fiber diets are recommended to help with constipation, but require sufficient fluid intake or they may make constipation worse.

Adequate fluid intake, or hydration, is especially important to consider for children who are unable to tolerate large-volume tube feedings.

Homemade blended formulas can be tailored to meet the child's fluid needs. Children on homemade blended diets can receive fluid through liquids used to prepare the formula—such as broths, milk, juices and wet foods—and from additional water given separately.

Children frequently need more fluid than they're able to receive from the homemade blended formula. This is particularly true when the homemade blended formula becomes thicker as it evolves to include more pureed food and less of the liquid formula.

Dehydration

When children take in insufficient fluid, or when they use up too much fluid without replacement, dehydration occurs. The water content of the body becomes too low.

Classical signs of acute dehydration include dry lips, nose or mouth; flushed skin; increased heart rate; constipation; lethargy; migraine headaches and even tiredness, weakness or confusion. If the child is not urinating regularly or has dark-colored, strong-smelling urine, additional fluids are needed.

Although most medical and dietary focus is on preventing acute dehydration, the concept of chronic or ongoing dehydration also must be considered.

A theory of water management in the body by Fereydoon Batmanghelidj, M.D., suggests that water itself powers the pumping mechanism that allows individual cells to draw in water and become fully hydrated. He believes that this pumping mechanism also provides a substantial amount of energy to the body. Thus, adequate water is vital to the body's optimal functioning.

The cells of the body are 75 percent water. The brain is 85 percent water and is very sensitive to even the smallest amount of dehydration.

Batmanghelidj theorizes that when even a small deficiency in water is present, the body shifts into a "drought-management system" which can lead to chronic dehydration. Neurotransmitters appear to ration the water that is available, directing it away from less vital parts of the body and into the brain and other essential organs.

Feeling thirsty and having a dry mouth aren't the most important signals that the body needs water. These signals kick in when the body already has lost enough cellular fluid to trigger the initial stages of chronic dehydration, and has begun to ration fluids.

Thirst signals are often unclear to children and adults who are chronically dehydrated, as well as those who receive their nourishment through feeding tubes.

Often the last signal of dehydration is a dry mouth. The body can suffer from dehydration even though the mouth is moist.

Gastrointestinal pain and discomfort can be major signals that the body is not getting enough water. Inadequate water in the gastrointestinal system may result in inefficient digestion, delayed stomach emptying and increased constipation.

For these reasons, it's essential to provide additional water in the diet of children receiving homemade blended formulas, and not to rely on the child's request for water as an indicator of dehydration.

Fluid Requirements

Parents and caregivers often are surprised to learn how great a volume of liquid children need. Sometimes children will ask for drinks and can tell parents when they're thirsty; more often, children need help to make sure they meet their fluid needs. This is especially true for tube fed children.

Fluid requirements can be determined using the following table, which provides recommendations based on weight. The numbers shown here are higher than traditional medical recommendations that are based on basic water needs for metabolism.

Recommended Amounts of Daily Fluids	
Child's Weight	Total 24-Hour Fluid Needs
7 lbs	2 cups (16 fluid ounces)
12 lbs	3.5 cups (28 fluid ounces)
21 lbs	5 cups (40 fluid ounces)
26 lbs	6 cups (48 fluid ounces)
36 lbs	7 cups (56 fluid ounces)
44 lbs	8 cups (64 fluid ounces)
63 lbs	9.5 cups (76 fluid ounces)
99 lbs	10.5 cups (84 fluid ounces)
119 lbs	10.5 cups (84 fluid ounces)

Adapted from Lucas B. (ed.) Children with Special Health Care Needs - Nutrition Care Handbook. American Dietetic Association, Chicago, IL. 2004 (page 106)

Too much fluid also can cause problems. The kidneys of an infant are immature and babies from birth to 12 months are more vulnerable to developing fluid over-load. Check with the child's physician before adding extra water for a child less than 1 year of age. Children who have cardiac, renal, liver or respiratory conditions may need to have their fluids restricted. The child's healthcare team must be consulted when there are special medical conditions, and they will determine the amount of fluid that is safe and appropriate.

Children need a balance of fluids provided throughout the day. Fluid can be provided within the blended formula and separately (free water) as "between meal," or "pre-meal" boluses. The ultimate water amounts and presentation methods may differ for each child.

Fluid improves texture and helps the formula move through the tube, but it's essential to balance fluid and nutrient needs. Too little fluid in a blended formula makes it difficult-to-impossible to move it through the tube. But when parents mix too much fluid with the child's homemade blended formula, it takes a lot more to achieve the recommended calorie and nutrient goals. This is a concern for tube fed children who have trouble comfortably handling volume.

Many families have found that broths, milks and juices work well for the fluid component of blended meals, and water can be given separately through the post-meal water flushes, between-meal water "snacks" or pre-meal water bolus "drinks" given through the tube 20 to 30 minutes prior to a meal.

Many parents and therapists have found that offering a water bolus 30 minutes prior to the tube meal supports both the greater fluid needs of a child receiving thicker food-based formula and improves the child's volume tolerance. The gastrointestinal system requires a large amount of fluid to support efficient breakdown of food in the stomach and for the pancreas to create a neutralizing watery fluid that supports the digestion of food.

Some professionals caution parents against giving water during the day because they believe it fills up the child and inhibits taking needed calories in the formula or food. This, however, is not true. Unlike food, water doesn't have to be digested and generally moves through the gastrointestinal tract rapidly. Within 30 minutes it usually has left the stomach and been absorbed by the small intestine. The added water in the body then is able to support the entire gastrointestinal system

and digestion. When water is given through the tube 30 minutes prior to a meal, it typically has left the stomach when the tube feeding is given.

Initially, the water bolus should be an amount the child can handle without discomfort 100 percent of the time. This amount is increased by 15 mls or ccs (i.e., ½ oz.) over a period of weeks and months, until the child is comfortable with a six- to eight-ounce bolus given within a five to ten minute period. The goal is to provide a sense of fullness without pain and discomfort.

Because the stomach is now filling and emptying relatively rapidly, bolus water feedings can build the child's awareness of positive feelings associated with stomach relaxation and expansion. This can result in the child's ability to accept larger bolus feedings of the formula and provide greater interest in eating orally.

Increased water also improves the efficiency of digestion, removes waste from the body, thins down mucus and reduces congestion and gagging. Each of these factors contributes to positive associations with both tube feeding and oral feeding.

Careful with Amounts!

It must be noted that if the body receives too much water, it may be unable to handle the volume of fluid efficiently. In the process of urinating large amounts of fluid, the kidneys can pull essential minerals such as sodium (salt) from the body. This fluid overload or water intoxication, though rare, can cause seizures and other neurological problems. Your child's healthcare team can help you determine individual fluid and sodium needs.

For additional information on the theory of chronic dehydration and the body's need for water see:

Batmanghelidj, F. (2003). *Your Body's Many Cries for Water.*
Falls Church, VA: Global Health Solutions.

Batmanghelidj, F. (2003). *Water for Health, for Healing, for Life.*

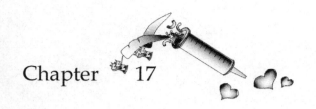

Chapter 17

Ongoing Dietary Support

Jude Trautlein, R.D.

Children with feeding tubes can maximize their nutrient intake using homemade blended formulas. To ensure this, families need continued support from both the primary care physician and a registered dietitian (R.D.) who works with children. Ideally, the dietitian will have had experience with tube feedings and blended formulas.

Registered dietitians are professionals who translate the science of nutrition into everyday information about food. They're uniquely trained to work with and advise the general public and people with special dietary needs about nutrition, food and diet.

An R.D. assesses each child's individual nutrient needs and ensures those needs are being met. The child's age, weight, medical condition, food allergies, medication use, and social and cultural background all help the R.D. determine optimal diet composition.

Unfortunately, children often leave a hospital on a tube feeding regimen with no plan for nutritional follow-up. As they grow and mature, their nutrient needs change. Those receiving nutrition via tube need to be monitored to ensure they continue to meet their protein, fluid, fiber and micronutrient needs for optimal growth and energy.

Most families start by providing a commercial formula to their tube fed child. When they initiate a change to a homemade blended formula, the R.D. can advise which foods to begin with, relating them to the child's health status, medication use and growth needs. Slowly adding new foods allows families to assess tolerance and allows the child's gastrointestinal tract to become accustomed to variety. As each new food is added to the diet, the R.D. can advise about additional changes needed to meet the child's nutrient needs.

Close follow-up is essential to make sure the child is receiving adequate fluids and adjusting to the volume of formula necessary for proper nutrition. Weekly or monthly sessions with the R.D. should continue until the transition to a homemade blended formula is complete and the child is accepting homemade food and growing appropriately. Children should be evaluated more often if they experience any difficulties, including inability to tolerate volume, weight loss, gastrointestinal discomfort, medication changes, vomiting or diarrhea.

As children grow older their nutrient needs continue to change and it's important to address these needs by altering the homemade blended formula accordingly.

An R.D. also is a valuable resource when children transition to oral feeding. At any point, an R.D. can analyze the nutritional adequacy of a child's diet and provide recommendations.

Ideally children will have follow-up visits with an R.D. every six months. Once the child is growing appropriately and is medically stable, this may change to annual monitoring.

For more information on finding a registered dietitian in your area contact:
The American Academy of Nutrition and Dietetics at (800) 877-1600
or online at http://www.eatright.org

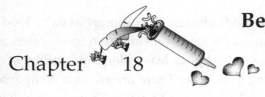

Chapter 18

Beginning a Homemade Blended Diet:
Where to Start

Ellen Duperret, R. D.
Marsha Dunn Klein, M.Ed., OTR/L

With support from your child's pediatrician, you've decided to tiptoe into the continuum of homemade blended formulas. One of the first questions asked is, what's THE recipe?

Actually there's not "THE" recipe. It's an evolving recipe, an evolving diet. The blend is individual for each child and family. It's developed through the same slow process that's used with orally fed children who are transitioning from breast milk or formula to foods.

When parents first introduce rice cereal and strained foods to their orally fed child, they proceed at a rate the child can handle. They respond to the child's reactions to flavor and texture, and to how well the new food is tolerated by the child's system. If all goes well and the new food is enjoyed, parents respond by offering more with enthusiasm. But if the child is very cautious or has an adverse reaction, then parents will respond more cautiously.

Parents don't know on that first day of food introduction what the actual diet or "recipe" will be when their child is eighteen months old or two years old. They just start. The child's diet evolves from a blend of information about the child's responses and ability to master new skills, and the parent's knowledge about balanced nutrition. The pediatrician monitors weight and growth and, when all goes well, the diet continues to expand. If the child has adverse reactions to particular foods or has difficulty growing as expected, then the plan is modified by parents with input from physicians or dietitians.

This same pattern is followed when introducing a homemade blended formula to a tube fed child. You just start, not knowing what the final blended formula diet or "recipe" will be. It's not yet known if the child ultimately will be given only one or two foods to supplement commercial formula or breast milk, or will be able to handle more. Those decisions are difficult to make with limited information. Parents first must find out how their child responds to each new food, what foods are tolerated, what foods interest the child, and the amount of calories and volume the child can handle.

Most families start the homemade blended formula process as they do with their orally fed children. They just start, introducing one food and building from there.

What Kind of Feeding Tube?

Homemade blended formulas seem to be easiest with catheter tubes with a diameter of 14 French or greater or with most sizes of button-type (gastrostomy) tubes that end in the stomach.

Some families have had success introducing small amounts of baby food thinly diluted with formula into the smaller nasogastric tubes (typically 5-8 French diameter) but it would be difficult to transition to a complete homemade blended formula with such a small tube. The volume would need to be quite large because purees need to be very dilute to pass through these tiny tubes.

Homemade blended formulas were initially not recommended to be put through tubes that end in the jejunum at the top of the small intestine (J-tubes). Only specialized "predigested" or more broken down, more easily digested formulas, were recommended. Recently, some families and dietitians have had more experience using regular formulas directly into the jejunum and have introduced some homemade blended food carefully. It must be remembered that the stomach is designed to expand with a meal. The small intestine is designed as a tube for transport and further digestion. It's not meant to take in a bolus or meal. Any attempt to use the jejunum for homemade blended food feedings *must* involve *medical permission* as well as very slow presentation and small volumes. Rapid presentation of large volumes in a tube that does not expand can cause negative gastrointestinal reactions and considerable discomfort.

Some people have successfully tiptoed into the introduction of simple purees to children with GJ-tubes (gastro-jejeunal tubes). They use the jejeunal tube to give the special commercial formula (such as Neocate Jr®., Alimentum®, Vivonex®) and then, as the child's system settles down, vomiting decreases and the child begin to grow, tiny amounts of easy-to-digest puree are sometimes introduced into the gastrostomy port of the GJ-tube. This must be done in conjunction with the child's medical team support.

What Foods to Try First?

For orally fed children, pediatricians usually recommend offering rice cereal and vegetables and fruits first, one at a time.

Rice cereal often is a first food because it provides supplemental iron that's especially needed by breast-fed babies in the second half of the first year of life. If your child is offered only breast milk through the tube, ask your pediatrician whether more iron through rice cereal or some other supplement is necessary. But, because most commercial formulas for tube fed babies and toddlers already have iron in them, rice cereal isn't as necessary as a first blended food, so parents of tube fed children are usually free to pick a vegetable or fruit to begin.

Orally fed babies often are offered strained foods in a sequence of easy-to-digest yellow vegetables or non-citrus fruits, and then green vegetables. This sequence isn't set in stone, but should be a general guideline.

Simple foods chosen by commercial baby food companies for stage one and two foods often are the easiest to digest, least allergenic and most pleasing to babies. There are reasons companies don't make baby food kale, cabbage, artichokes, green peppers or asparagus for their first foods!

In our experience, families pick easy first foods such as carrots, sweet potatoes, squash, applesauce, banana, pears, apricots, papaya, guava, peaches or mango. Families often use stage one and two foods available in the baby food section of grocery stores as starter foods, or make their own variation by blending a homemade version. Either way, the initial introduction is a single food and not a combination of foods.

The most efficient first foods are thinly pureed commercial baby foods. They tend to flow through the tube most easily and have a known number of calories per ounce. Parents want to have success in these first offerings, and they want their children to succeed. They want to know the volume and calories, how carefully the food has been prepared and how their child responds. Families don't want to invest in special blenders or special foods until they get a sense that a homemade blended formula will work for their child. Parents, of course, can make their own foods from the start, and many do so with great success.

Common First Foods

Vegetables	Carrots, Squash, Sweet potatoes
Fruits	Applesauce, Pears, Apricots Bananas, Papaya, Mango Peach, Plums

How Much at First?

Offer a small amount of pureed food in the tube at first. Remember, this whole process is one of tiptoeing! The amount that's right for one child isn't necessarily right for another.

Some children have been eating orally along with their tube feedings, or have been taking a food-based formula, such as Compleat® Pediatric. Their parents may have more confidence because the child is handling some real foods already.

However, many children with feeding tubes have a very sensitive gastrointestinal system, or a low tolerance for any change in the mealtime routine, or little to no experience with any foods other than formula. The child's history may be that even small changes in the diet lead to vomiting or discomfort.

The general rule of thumb is to try *with caution* and add more later. Most parents start with either one-half or one ounce of thinly pureed baby foods once a day, adding more if it's well accepted.

With orally fed children, a couple of small baby spoons of pureed food is usually given at first, NOT a quarter of a cup of the new food! And just because orally fed babies have a teaspoon of something today doesn't mean their systems will handle a cup of it tomorrow. It's easy to be very excited about the introduction of purees and want to give whole syringes of pureed food right away. But remember, it takes a while for orally fed children to increase their food volume, as their digestive systems become more efficient and stomach capacities increase. In the same way, tube fed children need time to get used to the initial food and provide sufficient feedback that it's being well tolerated.

Additionally, many tube fed children are volume sensitive. Parents often tell us their child can take a certain amount of formula in a certain number of minutes. They have the timing and volume planned out exactly for each meal in order to give the maximum calories with the fewest negative reactions. Many parents worry that introducing blended foods may upset this refined balance.

That's exactly why we suggest beginning slowly, watching volume and duration carefully. The volume is the amount of the bolus meal (in mls, ccs, or ounces) and the duration is the time needed to complete the tube feeding meal.

Some pureed baby foods are thin and others are thick. (Baby food bananas, for example, are much thicker than baby food pears.) This affects how the food mixes with the formula as well as how it influences the final bolus volume. For example, adding an ounce of pureed pears to a four-ounce bolus doesn't add a full ounce of overall volume. The pears mix with the formula and thicken it. It does increase the volume somewhat, but not by an ounce. Many children can handle a small increase in volume, especially if it's provided over a slightly longer period of time. Increasing the meal duration can provide just enough extra time for the child's digestive system to respond to the increased volume.

When volume is a difficult issue for a child, a small amount of puree can be given while lowering the formula volume slightly, so that the addition of the puree doesn't change the total volume. But often the number of calories in an ounce of pureed fruits or vegetables is slightly less than the number of calories in an ounce of plain formula, especially if the formula already is highly concentrated. If only one food is added to a single bolus each day, this may not amount to a significant reduction in calories or nutrients. If there's concern about overall calories, many families find a time later in the day to add the formula calories back into the total daily intake.

Try It Yourself!

- Add one ounce of a thin pureed food to eight ounces of formula. Measure exactly: notice the volume increase.

- Add one ounce of a thick pureed food to eight ounces of formula. Notice how the density of the added food changes the final volume.

When to Offer the New Food in the Daily Routine?

A child's first foods can be offered mixed in with a commercial formula or breast milk meal, or given between meals as a "snack."

Many families choose to offer a little pureed food at mealtime by mixing a small amount of puree with the formula bolus and watching for a reaction. Tube feedings can be time consuming and, for many, the thought of adding yet another feeding can be a bit overwhelming. Mixing pureed food with the feeding does increase the volume and change the caloric density. Combining it with the commercial formula has the advantage of thinning the puree so it's more easily pushed through the tube. Some children handle the combination well however, for others, it can be uncomfortable.

Some families prefer to give a tiny bolus of a plain food, with no formula, so that during burps the child might experience a small "taste" that's not flavored by the formula. Liquid may need to be added to the puree to thin it to the point where it flows easily through the syringe. Many parents use water or nectars as a "thinner" initially, until they're more confident about the child's ability to handle foods.

Other families use a combination. They start by offering a new food in the formula and then gradually, as they that see their child is tolerating it well, they separate out the food and then give it as a snack.

How to Offer the Food?

Both purees and formula mixed with pureed food are thicker than plain commercial formula, and most parents indicate they're more easily delivered through thicker diameter "bolus" extensions or thicker catheter tubes, rather than the tinier formula or pump extensions. Most families who have been providing drip pump or gravity drip feedings usually initiate syringe feedings with the plunger for these early

homemade meals. The rate they deliver the food depends on the child's tolerance of volume.

There are some families who have had success giving a very thin homemade formula more slowly from a gravity feeding bag or feeding pump. This seems to work for children who are being fed a very small amount of blended food mixed with commercial formula, or a thinned puree without formula. It also seems to work for children who receive the feeding in a mealtime bolus of two hours or less. A homemade blended formula that's too thick will just clog the pump.

Parents can use a feeding pump bag that has an ice pouch so the formula is kept chilled. But feeding a homemade blended formula over an extended time period (more than an hour or overnight feeding) is not recommended because of the increased possibility of food contamination.

Signs of Food Tolerance

What are the signs that an orally fed child is tolerating a new food? Those same signs apply for tube fed children receiving homemade blended formulas. The child enjoys the food, has no rash, no vomiting, no diarrhea, no constipation and no irritability. Though it's not uncommon for the child's bowel movements to change in consistency with the introduction of pureed foods, significant changes in these areas may be cause to question tolerance.

Food Progression

As children demonstrate that they can handle their first foods with no adverse reactions, the amounts given in a day can be increased by:

- Adding the same small amount of the puree to more than one bolus.

- Increasing the volume of the puree at a meal or snack.

When all goes well with this first food, consider offering another new food, following the same slow, cautious, observant sequence.

How does a parent decide which food to introduce next? The main thing to remember is to try only one new single food at a time, and not a combination of foods. This allows you to rule out allergies and check for tolerance before moving on. If too many new foods are introduced at once, parents won't know which food wasn't tolerated, or which food caused an allergic reaction.

Once the child has shown that several single purees are accepted well by the body, those single foods can be combined in various meals.

Calorie Adjustment

For orally fed children, the amount of breast milk or formula is reduced as the child eats more by mouth. Often a child will make the adjustment themselves by having less interest in the breast or bottle.

When tube fed children can handle a number of separate single foods in greater volume, there also needs to be an adjustment in the quantity of commercial formula or breast milk offered. Because parents have control over how much is put into the tube, they will need to be sensitive to their child's cues of fullness and not push the calorie totals to the point where the child is vomiting because of being too full.

Families estimate the total number of formula calories the child receives by tube during the day and night by multiplying the ounces by the calories per ounce. For example:

Formula Fed Child
        24 ounces of formula in the day
        x 30 calories per ounce = total daily calorie
                                count of 720 cals.

Breast Milk Fed Baby
        24 ounces of breast milk per day
        x 20 calories (average) per ounce
                                = total daily calorie
                                count of 480 cals.

Some children can handle receiving the same amount of liquid formula along with the added puree, and the puree calories become "extra" calories that can boost growth. Gradually however, some of the formula will need to be reduced as puree volume increases. The formula quantity initially may be reduced one ounce at a time as the child takes in each ounce of puree, but as the puree amounts increase, there will need to be a recalculation of vitamins and nutrients to ensure optimum overall nutrition.

Tolerance is certainly an indicator that the child is moving in the right direction with the addition of purees, but the most important indicator of calorie needs is overall growth. Any child who is on tube feedings, and ANY tube fed child being transitioned into some form of homemade blended formula, should have height and weight monitored regularly.

"THE" Recipe

Once the introductory stage is passed, families are encouraged to develop a daily meal plan for their own child based on solid principles of pediatric nutrition. Guidelines for designing a daily meal plan are shared in other chapters of this handbook. These guidelines are based on each child's nutritional and energy needs. Some families develop a standard recipe structure that allows for variation and dietary diversity. Others change the "menu" daily. Still others evolve to a comfort level where they confidently blend the family meal and provide that through the tube. Families of tube fed children have shared recipes that blend well as a starter, but no one recipe is THE recipe that works for all children of all ages and with different energy needs.

When creating a recipe, we strongly suggest working with a registered dietitian to analyze the nutritional components of the recipe in detail— calories, fluid, macronutrients and micronutrients.

The "recipe" is only a starting point. A physician and/or dietitian can help with individualized nutrition. Putting a combination of foods in the tube is where many parents get creative, adding special foods, supplements, herbs and spices. Working with dietitians and integrative medicine physicians, many families have discovered special foods or supplements that improve their child's health. Some families, in working with their dietitians and physicians, have found that adding extras such as omega-3 fatty acids, probiotics, vitamins, calorie-boosting supplements or certain spices to the diet is helpful.

Finding "THE" recipe for a homemade blended diet is a journey in which parents use their ordinary knowledge of feeding children, their intuition about their child's reaction to each dietary change, and input from the medical team regarding growth, development, and medical issues, in order to do what it takes for their child to succeed.

For additional information on progressions in tube feedings and formulas see:

Klein, M.D. (2007). Tube Feeding Transition Plateaus. *Exceptional Parent Magazine*, 36:06 (February).

For additional information on building an individualized homemade blended formula see:

Klein, M.D. and Morris, S.E. (2007). Chapter 25 – Anatomy of a Recipe. *Homemade Blended Formula Handbook*. Tucson, AZ: Mealtime Notions, LLC.

Klein, M.D. and Morris, S.E. (2007). Chapter 26 – Core Guidelines for a Homemade Blended Formula. *Homemade Blended Formula Handbook*. Tucson, AZ: Mealtime Notions, LLC.

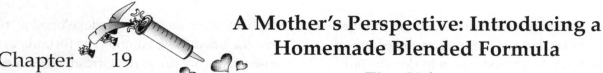

A Mother's Perspective: Introducing a Homemade Blended Formula

Tina Valente

"Homemade formula? Why in the world would you want to go to so much trouble when you can just pop open a can?"

That's the response I've gotten from a number of people, most notably doctors and dietitians. My reasons are numerous for feeding my gastrostomy tube fed child a diet primarily made up of homemade formula. The most important reason, in my mind, is that it has given me a more active role in my child's diet and nutrition.

Introducing homemade formula has had numerous rewards, but both patience and flexibility are needed for a successful experience.

My son Joey, nine, has a genetic liver disease. He also has a number of gastrointestinal issues that complicate his life, including severe reflux, slow stomach emptying and malabsorption of fats and vitamins. Eating has been difficult since birth and Joey was soon classified as "failure to thrive." At seven months he received a nasogastric tube for supplemental feedings, and a more permanent gastrostomy tube at 9 months. He was prescribed a special easily digested formula and placed on a "feeding schedule." As he grew older and his dietary needs changed, he was prescribed a variety of canned formulas made by commercial formula companies.

Joey has had continual feeding therapy over the years to promote his oral skills and improve his relationship with food. Unfortunately, it became obvious after a few years that it was unlikely Joey would grow out of his reflux and gastrointestinal issues as everyone had hoped. Currently he eats some foods orally, though the majority of his nutrition continues to be supplied by his tube.

The first routine established for Joey's nutrition was very mechanical and became rather depressing for our family. We pumped commercial canned formula into our son as prescribed, yet we felt that both his health and emotional well-being could be better served. Despite the great amounts of formula he was receiving, his growth and weight gain was very slow.

Additionally, we felt that he wasn't always included in the family aspect of food preparation and mealtime. When we did have him join us at the table, the food he was served most often wasn't even touched. This "wasting" of food was particularly difficult for me to see and it amplified my sense of depression. Like most moms, I envisioned baking cookies and making special meals for my child. I felt cheated out of that aspect of my relationship with my son.

Apparently I was not alone. Our occupational therapist started a tube feeding support group for parents looking to improve their children's lives. The initial focus of this group was to investigate homemade formulas as an option for our children's nutrition. The group included parents of tube fed children, feeding specialists, dietitians and, eventually, a pediatrician. We read about and met other parents who'd had success with homemade blended formulas. I became convinced it could be beneficial for our son and decided to take the plunge. I soon discovered that a very methodical approach was needed when introducing a homemade formula. Preparation and research were also required.

The first step was to discuss the idea of homemade formulas with Joey's doctors and his feeding team. At the time, Joey was 3 years old and his health status was fairly stable. Many of his doctors had a hard time understanding why I would want to work so hard when canned formula was so easy. Others were concerned that he wouldn't get adequate nutrition and calories. But a few encouraged me, believing that there were benefits in a varied diet of fresh foods that couldn't be obtained from a can.

I made appointments with a dietitian familiar with Joey's particular dietary and health needs and together we developed a plan to slowly start incorporating fresh foods into Joey's diet. We reviewed his caloric and nutritional needs and calculated the calories per ounce required for his homemade formula. Total daily water requirements also were reviewed. After all our research was complete, we then asked the doctors to review our plan and give their approval. With approval and a plan in hand, I slowly started adding new foods to Joey's diet. I approached each new addition carefully and only added one new food at a time. I started by adding some jarred baby foods. Peaches were chosen as our first addition. In a blender, we added jarred baby food peaches to his canned formula to make a smoothie that easily went through his tube. Initially, we just gave Joey two ounces of the homemade mixture with one meal. Slowly we increased the amount of mixture to two ounces at every meal. I continued to add peaches for five days until I was sure his system could tolerate the change. I then tried a vegetable (baby food carrots) and again tried that food for five days.

Each new ingredient added to Joey's formula was slowly incorporated in this manner. Luckily, Joey's system was very tolerant of the changes and he didn't have any problems adapting to the new diet. As we progressed, we were able to increase the amount of homemade formula that he received at each meal.

Because the addition of any purees to canned formula thickens it, we soon realized we needed to use the syringe to present the pureed food instead of the pump. Not only did the thicker puree not move well through the pump, but we also were concerned about it staying fresh. We wanted to eliminate the chance of food spoilage.

We moved along cautiously, adding new individual foods and new food combinations. Within a few months, we began replacing the baby foods with fresh fruits and vegetables. Later, with the help of his dietitian, we developed a "recipe" that included some commercial formula as the base of the diet, fresh fruit, fresh vegetables, whole grains, baby food meats, milk, yogurt and an oil for additional fat and calories. We inched our way up to increased volumes during daytime meals and analyzed and re-analyzed our blends, all the time watching Joey's growth patterns with his medical team. We continued to individualize Joey's diet based on HIS reactions. We knew each child's tolerance for solid foods or calories per ounce varied and we were pleased that Joey's system seemed very well suited for these gradual changes.

As Joey slowly tolerated bigger amounts, his daytime feeding routine began to resemble the mealtime schedule of children his age who eat by mouth. We worked his schedule into three or four large bolus meals, with additional little snacks and water boluses during the day, and then supplemented at night as needed with canned formula by pump. Eventually we eliminated all night feedings when we were sure he could grow and handle the bigger volumes needed during the day.

We began developing our own "recipe" and our own variations on that "recipe." After we had added some basic vegetables and fruits one at a time, we decided next to prepare grains as a congee. We had learned that a congee is a traditional Chinese breakfast porridge most often made from slow cooked rice and water. The term also can be used to describe slow cooked grain or millet. It's said that the longer congee is cooked, the more powerful it becomes. It's an ingredient that is easily incorporated into a homemade formula diet as a good source of grains. Because the grains are cooked for such a long time, they're very easily digested. We used 12-grain cereal, short grain brown rice, millet and quinoa. We added various spices to the cooking process, such as ginger and cloves, as we read they can provide stomach-soothing properties for some children. They also fill the house with comforting aromas as the congee cooks.

We got creative and more confident as we prepared vegetables for Joey's blended meals. We started with store-bought baby food vegetables but gradually expanded to homemade versions of family favorites such as green beans, corn, broccoli, carrots, sweet potatoes, squash and peas. We later added asparagus, avocados and spinach. As we continued to read about nutrition and discuss diet with team members, we learned about the richness of vitamins and minerals in vegetables that typically had not been on our regular family menu, such as cabbage, kale, Brussels sprouts and beets. We decided to cook some of these vegetables in our slow cooker and add them to our evolving "recipe." (Of course we tried each vegetable individually to ensure Joey's tolerance before adding them to our blend.) We would coarsely chop and wash some combination of beets, spinach, kale, Brussels sprouts, red cabbage and carrots and cook them slowly in the cooker. Overtime, we added spices to these too. This blended mixture was added to our "recipe." Now, we use this slow cooked mixture as our vegetable base and blend it again with a fresh or frozen organic vegetable of our choice, to vary Joey's vegetable diet. By varying the vegetables with each batch, a different vegetable is being eaten every two days. By rotating and changing the vegetables, herbs and spices, a greater variety of necessary vitamins, nutrients and antioxidants can be included in our homemade diet.

Meats also started with commercial baby food. It was easy and the calories and purity of it were known. However, in an effort to prepare our own unique diet for Joey we decided to prepare our own meats too. We introduced one meat at a time to be sure it was tolerated. We ultimately used a slow cooker and our Vita-Mix high powered blender to make a variety of meat purees. We started with organic chicken, since we already had used baby food chicken in our previous recipe. We cooked the meats in a slow cooker with onions, garlic, herbs and spices.

Now we also occasionally substitute beans as a protein source and cook them in the same manner

as the meat. Beans may not be a suitable addition to the diets of children who may be affected by the gastrointestinal discomfort that can result, but Joey did well with them.

As time went on, we continued to investigate nutritional options for Joey. Our family consulted with dietitians, read articles and also consulted with a doctor specializing in pediatric integrative medicine. Joey's formula evolved and became less and less dependent on canned commercial formula. We gradually included some food supplements to round out the calorie and nutrient blend. We switched to a dairy-free diet on the recommendation of a consulting physician. This change seemed to help improve Joey's slow stomach emptying.

The results and pay-off that we've experienced have been phenomenal. The biggest improvements were almost immediate. Joey's weight gain and growth, which always had been markedly slow, dramatically improved. His height and weight had never registered on the growth charts. Within about six months of altering Joey's diet, he finally reached the fifth percentile. At his present age of nine, Joey is solidly at the 25th percentile for both height and weight.

Another immediate improvement was a new interest in oral foods. In our case, there was a direct correlation between the switch to home-made blended foods and Joey's willingness to try new food tastes and textures. He also seemed to take more interest and enjoyment in food preparation and eating with the family. Now we involve him in the preparation of the homemade formula and it's empowering for him to make some of the choices of what goes into the blender and eventually his stomach. He can decide if he wants peaches or pears, carrots or green beans, etc. He enjoys blending up food that's left on his plate. He has the satisfaction of feeling that he finished his meal like everyone else.

There's also an emotional benefit for the rest of the family. The sense of frustration I once felt about leftover food is gone. I have a new sense of control and pride in knowing that I'm providing my son with the very best nutrition possible. I feel that the time I spend making his blended formula is an investment in his health and his future.

We began this whole process nervously calculating calories, ounces and specific nutritional components of each meal. Gradually we began to relax and have confidence in our ability as parents to make meal-by-meal decisions for our son. We saw him growing and the pressure was off! We knew Joey was thriving and we saw that his friends' parents didn't worry about the exact components of every single meal. We felt pride that our child was getting Brussels sprouts, avocado, salmon and flax seed meal, and not chicken nuggets and French fries! Sometimes we now just blend the table foods we're eating with some of his formula. We offer him the family meal orally and let him eat what he wants, what feels good and tastes good to him. What he doesn't finish at the table is blended up and provided through his tube.

Through our journey, I've learned that flexibility is the key to successfully incorporating homemade formula into our lives. The process doesn't need to be an all-or-nothing proposition. There have been bumps in the road when Joey has been extremely ill or his reflux worsened. During those times, the commercial formula is easier for him to digest and we may rely upon it for much of his nutrition. There are also times when our lives are extremely hectic and I'll rely on commercial formula as the basis for Joey's nutrition and simply add fresh foods to it. It's also a convenient supplement to have on hand at school and is extremely easy to pack for travel or vacation.

Once I made the decision to start working toward homemade formula, I realized that it didn't have to completely replace commercial formula and that it wasn't a "failure" if we gave him some commercial formula. The percentage of a homemade blended formula that Joey receives on a daily basis varies depending upon his health and circumstances and we're all fine with that!

Today Joey is a happy, outgoing nine year old. He's in third grade and adapting well to the public school setting. He brings his snack and lunch to school like all the other kids. After eating what he can with his classmates, he goes to the nurse's office for a supplemental bolus feeding of his homemade blended formula as well as some commercial formula that I pack for him daily.

Both Joey and I have come to see his feeding tube as a blessing. When he's ill or his reflux is acting up, he'll sometimes ask to skip his oral meal and simply receive a bolus feeding. I have the peace of mind that no matter what he eats orally, he'll still receive excellent nutrition through his tube fed meals. He may well be the best-nourished nine year old I know! Preparing his homemade blended food has allowed me to make peace with the tube, as it has become my partner in providing the best nourishment for my child.

Joey's Recipes

Joey's Original Basic Non-Dairy Diet

2 ounces cooked meat or ¼ can of salmon
     or 1 egg
1 avocado
⅓ cup wheat germ
1 piece of fresh fruit
5 Tbsp MCT Oil
2 ounces aloe vera juice
4 ounces of vegetable (baby food or fresh)
6 ounces of tofu yogurt
1½ cup soy or rice milk (enriched)
1 ounce of tofu cream cheese
4 ounces juice (plum, papaya, wheat grass,
     carrot, etc.)
3 Tbsp soy powder
2 Tbsp soybean butter
½ cup granola
⅓ cup flax seed meal
2 scoops Ultracare for Kids®
5 cans Peptamen Jr® formula

This provides approximately six 12-ounce servings for Joey.

Revised Basic Non Dairy Diet

6-ounce jar homemade meat
6-ounce jar homemade congee
6-ounce jar homemade chicken broth
6-ounce jar homemade vegetable blend
       (cabbage, beets, kale, beans),
          or ½ cup fresh cooked vegetables
1 avocado
⅓ c. aloe vera juice
6 ounces tofu yogurt
2 scoops soy powder
2 scoops Ultracare for Kids™
4 ounces juice (plum, papaya, carrot,
        wheatgrass, etc.)
2 cans Peptamen Jr™ formula
Calcium supplement

(Approximately six 12-ounce servings)

Joey's Congee

In a small crock pot combine:
1 cup grain (12-grain meal, wild rice, millet, etc.)
3 cups filtered water
Optional spices : our choices are cinnamon,
       cloves, nutmeg, ginger, etc.

Cook in a slow cooker for six to eight hours on low, stirring occasionally. I let it cool and then transfer to clean six-ounce dishwasher-cleaned Mason jars. I put the lids on tight and store them in the refrigerator for up to two weeks.

I use congee as part of individual meals for Joey, or mix it in a larger recipe for a day's meals. When using congee as an ingredient blended up in Joey's homemade formula, I typically use ½ cup if making a daily batch of formula, and a full six-ounce jar for a larger batch. Or, I may mix some with fruit and yogurt and call it breakfast!

Joey's Vegetables

When choosing vegetables to incorporate into our homemade formula, I usually use fresh vegetables that I cook in the slow cooker. Frozen vegetables can also be used. They can be added to the blender straight from the freezer without defrosting.

In a small slow cooker combine:
1 bunch of well-washed coarsely chopped fresh vegetables such as red cabbage, kale, beets, spinach, Brussels sprouts and carrots.

I cover the vegetables with filtered water and add herbs and spices such as turmeric, cumin, parsley, oregano, onion, or garlic. I cook this mixture until very soft, then let it cool, blend and transfer to dishwasher-clean lidded six-ounce Mason jars. I typically use four ounces of these vegetables in a six-serving batch of homemade formula, or I use it as my base and blend an additional fresh-cooked vegetable with it and use a total of four ounces of that in a daily batch. I rotate the additional fresh vegetable every few days to vary the diet.

Joey's Meat and Broth

In large crock pot combine:
1 lb fresh meat such as fresh boneless chicken or turkey, fresh ground lamb or one cup of well-washed dried bean mixture. If using fresh boneless fish, considerably less cooking time is necessary.

Add herbs, vegetables and spices as desired
    such as:
       Bunch fresh parsley
       Bunch fresh basil
       Organic carrots, chopped (3 – 4)
       Organic celery, chopped (3 - 4)
       Chopped onion
       2 garlic cloves, chopped
       Chopped bell pepper
       Peeled and chopped fresh ginger

I mix and vary the choices of vegetables and herbs for variety. I cover the meat mixture with filtered water and cook on low in a slow cooker for 12 hours, then let it cool.

I remove the meat to the high powered blender. I strain the broth and place some in clean six-ounce lidded Mason jars for later use. I then blend the meat with a small amount of broth and place in clean six-ounce Mason jars. The remaining vegetables also may be blended or discarded. I store this in the refrigerator for one to two weeks.

Joey's Chamomile Tea

(Joey has two ounces three times a day before meals. This has helped him with tummy upset.)

Combine and simmer for 30 minutes:

1 quart filtered water

2 tsp cinnamon chips (or 1 tsp powdered cinnamon)

1 tsp licorice shavings (this was individually prescribed for Joey for his liver health. It is not for everyone!)

1 tsp cardamon seeds

1 ounce fresh sliced ginger

I remove this mixture from the heat and add six teaspoons of bulk chamomile tea and then let it steep for 30 minutes. I strain and divide the tea into two-ounce servings.

These recipes are made specifically for Joey with his own special nutritional needs and are not for all children. Check with your team.

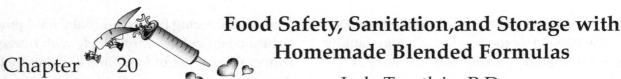

Chapter 20

Food Safety, Sanitation, and Storage with Homemade Blended Formulas

Jude Trautlein, R.D.

When preparing any food for our families, it's important to keep in mind safe food practices. We often don't think about food safety until a food related illness affects someone we know. Children under five years of age and those with chronic medical conditions are especially susceptible to food-borne illnesses. This must be kept in mind as families consider providing homemade blended formulas.

When using a commercial tube feeding formula, it's sufficient to store and transport the unopened containers at room temperature. But when preparing and providing homemade blended formulas for tube fed children, there are crucial safeguards that must be practiced to avoid food-borne illnesses.

It's impossible to know by sight, smell or taste if food has been contaminated with dangerous bacteria. The Partnership for Food Safety Education advocates using the following four steps to ensure the safety of food prepared at home: clean, separate, cook and chill.

Clean

Keeping hands and work surfaces clean is the first step to ensuring safe food. To wash hands effectively, rub them together with soap and warm water for at least 20 seconds, working the soap under the fingernails. Rinse under warm water and dry with a paper towel.

Washing kitchen surfaces and utensils in hot soapy water will alleviate disease-causing bacteria. Cutting boards can be cleaned by running them through the dishwasher. Many families use a disinfectant or diluted bleach solution to sanitize kitchen surfaces, towels and sponges. Paper towels, used once and then placed in the garbage, are a good way to help stop the spread of bacteria in the kitchen. Clean all utensils well after use.

Follow the cleaning directions for your specific blender. Vita-Mix, for example, recommends that their high powered blender, not be washed in a dishwasher as the detergent is harsh on the seals that protect the bearings. The manufacturer recommends filling it with warm water, adding one drip of dish soap and then running on high speed for 30 seconds.

The first step in preparing fresh vegetables and fruits is rinsing under running water and scrubbing away any dirt. Any bruises or marred areas must be cut off prior to using the produce.

Separate

Using separate cutting surfaces for raw meat, poultry and seafood reduces the potential for cross contaminating other foods. Having different colored cutting boards for each specific food type is a tip that's used by commercial kitchens. Never put cooked food in a container that's been used to hold raw food.

Cook

Cooking foods thoroughly will destroy bacteria. Using a clean food thermometer is the best way to ensure that foods are cooked to a safe temperature. Most foods are done at 165°F (74°C), however whole poultry should be heated to 180°F (83°C) and chicken breasts to 170°F (77°C).

Chill/Freeze

Keeping food cold keeps it safe. Never leave food or a homemade blended formula at room temperature for more than two hours. Using a thermometer will help determine if refrigerator temperatures remain below 40°F (4.5°C). Prompt refrigeration of perishable foods and leftovers is a healthy habit. Hot foods will chill more rapidly if placed in shallow containers before refrigerating. Homemade batches of puree should be used immediately, chilled in the refrigerator or frozen. Freezers should be kept at 0°F (- 18°C).

Common methods that parents use for freezing pureed foods are ice cube trays and individual-serving-size containers. A standard ice cube tray holds one-and-a-half to two tablespoons per cube. (This is the equivalent of about ¾ -1 an ounce per cube depending on how full you make it.) Check out your own ice cube tray to be sure of the actual quantity it holds to provide more specific information. This is helpful information as you calculate amounts for meals.

Ice Cube Tray Method

Pour the puree into a well-washed ice cube tray. Freeze. Pop out the cubes into a dated and labeled airtight freezer bag. Expel as much air as possible when closing the freezer bag. Consider using smaller freezer bags, such as quart-size bags rather than gallon size. You will use up the smaller bag more quickly and have less air exposure.

Individual-Serving-Size Containers

Pour puree into a well-washed single-serving-size container with an airtight lid. Expel as much air as possible when closing the lid.

Freezer Storage

The USDA (U.S. Department of Agriculture) recommends using frozen baby food purees in up to one month. We've reviewed a number of different resources about freezing fruits and vegetables, freezing meats, freezing common foods and freezing homemade baby food purees. Published guidelines vary widely with freezer temperature, types of foods and whether they're in the natural state or pureed. Many allow for longer freezer storage periods.

The USDA recommendation is more conservative than some others, but it makes sense when all the factors are taken into consideration, such as the daily opening and closing of the freezer (influencing constancy of freezer temperature), multiple openings of freezer bags, the combinations of foods prepared as homemade blended foods, and the fact that generally we're following the recommendations for preparing homemade baby food.

Helpful Freezing Hints from Parents

Grains can be tricky to freeze, thaw and put through the tube. The defrosted grains can be difficult to re-blend. Rice is an example of a food that seems to work best fresh. Many families find it's better to prepare smaller amounts and refrigerate for a few days rather than trying to freeze. If it must be frozen, freeze before blending, and blend it at the time of use.

Families preparing homemade blended formulas report that when several types of foods are mixed together (for example, meats, grains, vegetables, fruits, dairy and oils) and then frozen, the thawed mixture may not go through the tube as easily. It may be better to freeze individual types of food and mix or blend them together after thawing. By using the ice cube method, you can easily create your own combinations.

Milk or formula should be added at time of final blending for presentation. Formula manufacturers

For additional information see:

Fight Bac: Partnership for Food Safety Education: http://www.fightbac.org/main.cfm

Home Prepared Baby Food–USDA Resource: http://www.fns.usda.gov/tn/Resources/feedinginfants-ch12.pdf

FoodSafety.gov   Gateway to Government Food Safety Information: http://www.foodsafety.gov

Food Safety and Inspection Service: http://www.foodsafety.gov

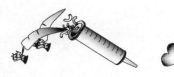

Storage Safety Summary

If Serving at Once	Serve freshly cooked and blended purees shortly after preparation. Do not let freshly cooked or thawed purees stand at room temperature, or between 40-140°F (4.5-60°C) for more than two hours. Serve boluses of homemade food in less than two hours. For extra safety, consider keeping the un-served portion of the bolus chilled. If using a pump for a bolus, offer it in less than two hours.
Refrigerator Storage	Maintain refrigerator temperature of 40°F (4.5°C). Keep formula in refrigerator until just before feeding. If transporting, use a thermal bag with ice or a cold pack. Store cooked strained fruits and vegetables and grains 2-3 days in clean, covered serving dishes in the refrigerator. Store strained meats for a day in the refrigerator. Store meat and vegetable combinations for 1-2 days in the refrigerator. Throw out food left out at room temperature for over two hours. Defrost frozen foods in the refrigerator.
Freezer Storage	Keep the freezer at a steady temperature of 0°F (- 18°C). Store homemade baby food purees for up to one month in the freezer. Do not refreeze previously frozen foods unless you have cooked them first. As per manufacturer's recommendations, do not freeze commercial formula.

Adapted from USDA Recommendations

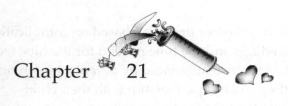

Chapter 21

Equipment to Support a Homemade Blended Formula

Marsha Dunn Klein, M.Ed., OTR/L

Families often ask what type of special equipment is necessary for providing a homemade blended diet for their child. The question has several different answers depending on the types of tubes, food delivery, types of food and complexity of the diet. Let's look at the child's tube feeding equipment and discuss how it works with homemade blended formulas, as well as the equipment that may be used in food preparation.

Types of Tubes

Although children can receive tube feedings by nasogastric and nasojejeunal tubes, most children who receive homemade blended formulas use either gastrostomy or jejeunal tubes. The diameter of these tubes can vary.

The nasogastric and nasojejeunal tubes pass through the nose into the stomach or jejeunum (top part of the small intestine). Because the tube goes through the nose, it must be narrow in diameter. Nasal tubes for infants and young children are typically 5 French to 8 French in diameter. ("French" is a unit of measure for tube sizes. The higher the number, the bigger the tube diameter.)

Gastrostomy tubes place food directly into the stomach and can be either catheter or button feeding tubes. These tubes are typically smaller in young infants (10, 12 or 14 French). Their size is increased to 16, 18 and 20 French as children grow.

The use of a homemade blended formula with nasogastric tubes is limited for several reasons. First of all, nasogastric tubes are traditionally used for short-term nutritional support. Physicians often recommend nasal tubes as part of a diagnostic workup to see if the child can grow while receiving supplementation, or to help the child put on weight while preparing for surgery, or to improve nutrient intake while trying to better understand the challenges the child is having with

growth and gastrointestinal function. They usually don't recommend homemade formulas as an added variable for an infant in the middle of multiple medical challenges requiring the initial supplemental calories. Infants at this stage frequently receive trials of different formulas, presentation techniques, volumes and feeding rates, in hopes of discovering what works best. Adding pureed foods is another variable that further complicates medical problem-solving and is regularly discouraged.

Physicians have supported the very cautious introduction of some homemade formulas for some toddlers and older children who have nasogastric tubes and are medically stable. The challenge for families is that the tube is VERY narrow, requiring a very thin formula. Also, it's difficult to get enough calories in a small enough volume to provide for full nutritional needs. Some parents have successfully added a small amount of a diluted baby food mixed with breast milk or formula to expand dietary diversity and provide a gentle introduction to a first food.

When the feedings are going from the nose to the jejeunum, not only is the tube narrow, but the food is entering the digestive system past the stomach. It's bypassing the digestive processes of the stomach. Initially, dietitians and pediatricians tend to prescribe a predigested commercial formula in this situation. But on a case-by-case basis, some teams have had success with other types of formulas as well. The jejeunum isn't flexible and stretchable like the stomach and doesn't allow for large volumes. Feedings placed in the jejeunum must be delivered slowly and in small quantities, and must be reviewed with the physician and dietitian to determine appropriateness for each child.

Historically, gastrostomy tube feedings were provided through catheter feeding tubes. These tubes had a large diameter and most commonly were used before commercial formula became available and blended food was the standard for nutrition. As the technology of tube feeding advanced, tubes became smaller and button feeding tubes often replaced catheter tubes.

As families move from liquid commercial formula toward pureed diets, the thickness of the diet increases and so do the complications in the method of food delivery. Families consistently describe success in giving homemade blended formulas through 14 French catheter tubes or larger. Smaller catheter sizes—though possible for homemade blended formula—are more restrictive because of the increased fluid necessary for easy flow through the narrower tube. Increased fluid creates a larger volume of formula, which some children can't tolerate.

Most families seem to be having consistent success using homemade blended formulas with the button-type tubes of multiple sizes. The French diameter (14, 16, 18, etc.) refers to the diameter of the tube as it enters a child's abdomen. However the inner workings of most button feeding tubes are a standard size. This means that the home-made blended formulas must move through the same diameter tube within the button, whether it is 14, 16, 18 French diameter. The bolus extensions also tend to be a standard size whether the abdominal size increases or decreases. Tubes are constantly being researched and new designs are evolving. It's important to check on specifications of the child's personal tube, and ultimately combine family experience with what works for your child in terms of volume and consistency.

Food Delivery

Tube feedings are offered via gravity by syringe or feeding bag, via pressure through a syringe with a plunger, or through a feeding pump. The choice of syringe or pump sometimes is determined by the capacity and sensitivity of the child's stomach. Sometimes it's a decision based on the preference of the physicians in a particular geographic region. At other times, it's based on complications of feedings and the time needed for the tube fed meal. It's also influenced by parents' preferences, as they create a partnership with their child during the tube feeding mealtime.

A feeding pump offers the advantage of delivering the formula at a pre-set rate; it also can provide feedings very slowly. This works well for the child who has difficulty handling volume at a feeding, or who has easy gagging and vomiting with any change in the rate at which the food is given. Sometimes it's difficult for parents to give formula at a steady enough rate for the child to succeed, so the pump can be a great help.

On the other hand, the pump has some disadvantages. It can accentuate the feeling of "procedure" rather than "mealtime." It's often used for extended feedings, over hours, full days and nighttime. The pre-set delivery of the same amount of formula makes it difficult for parents to adjust amounts spontaneously, in response to their child's cues. It also doesn't prepare the gastrointestinal system for the more random timing and volume of food that's characteristic of oral feeding. This factor is important when the child becomes ready for weaning from the tube.

Another disadvantage of the pump for use with homemade blended formulas is that the formula needs to be thin enough to flow easily through the pump and not clog it. The food can't be as thick as it would be if given with the syringe. Because much thinner food is necessary by pump, the volume needed for daily nutritional needs increases and can become a problem for a child.

Parents who provide nutrition by pump have described some successes with homemade blended formulas when the drip meal is given over two hours or less. A challenge in giving a homemade blended formula is that it shouldn't sit out at room temperature longer than two hours because of the possibility of food spoilage or bacterial contamination.

General suggestions for using homemade blended formulas with feeding pumps include:

- Be sure the food is thin enough to flow easily and not clog the pump.
- Homemade food should not be at room temperature for longer than two hours.
- Use chill bags to keep the formula chilled during delivery. Chill bags are specially designed pump bags with an ice pouch or place to put an ice packet. They're available through feeding pump supply companies.

Most people providing homemade blended formulas do so with a 60 ml syringe with a plunger. The plunger allows the parent to provide the food in varying degrees of thickness, even when it doesn't flow easily with gravity. The parent can slowly push the food through the syringe, watching the child's reaction and adjusting the flow accordingly.

Some parents use a syringe without the plunger and let the formula flow into the stomach by raising the syringe high enough for gravity to empty it. A homemade blended formula needs to be quite thin for this approach, just as it does when using the pump.

Complexity of the Diet

There is a continuum of dietary complexity for homemade blended formulas. The family that predominantly uses a commercial formula, blending in a commercially prepared baby food once a day, will need much different equipment than the family that chooses to provide all nutrition from homemade sources. When a small amount of thin baby food fruit or vegetable is added to commercial formula, many families have found that they need only stir well with a fork or whisk. At this stage, many have found they don't even need a blender. The action of the plunger in the syringe can usually move the diluted mixture into the stomach.

The Blender

Most families have found that a blender is required. Often an inexpensive blender is used while blending formula plus commercial baby food, or simple fruits and vegetables.

Most families who decide to offer more textured foods, meats, grains and nuts and a larger percentage of food than formula have found that a high powered blender is needed. Families have used different blenders, but many have repeatedly recommended a high powered blender, such as the Vita-Mix or Blendtec, because of their proven ability to smoothly blend meats and varied whole food diets. Additionally, both companies have an active program to work with families of tube fed children to offer a discount when the blender is used to provide tube feedings with homemade blended formulas.

Food Preparation

To make homemade food, appropriate chopping, cooking, blending and storage equipment is needed. Be sure to use a cutting board that's easy to clean. Some foods are boiled or steamed in a pan with a lid. Others use a slow cooker over extended periods of time. Many families have found that slow cookers are very useful in preparing meats and grains.

To prepare nuts and seeds for easy addition to the puree, families have ground them in a coffee grinder before adding them to the mixture for blending. The grinder has been very helpful in reducing clogs.

Some families have resorted to straining blended foods to remove the texture that could lead to clogs. They might strain through a strainer, or a piece of cheesecloth. This certainly can help eliminate clogs, but reduces the fiber of the mixture. Generally, using a powerful blender will eliminate the need for straining.

Some families prepare the food and serve it immediately, with no need for storage. Others will make one or two days' worth of meals. These will need to be refrigerated until transferred to airtight storage containers or canning jars. Still others make meal components ahead of time and mix them together at the time of each meal. One of the most common ways to store a homemade blended formula is to put the food in ice cube trays and freeze individual portions for later use, storing them in resealable plastic bags. Families measure the amount held in the ice cube trays (usually ¾ to one ounce). They then can calculate calories per cube of each food. As they become comfortable with diet preparation, they can defrost and reblend cubes of one or two of the fruits, vegetables, meats and grains they use as the foundation for their child's meal. Desired liquids and non-freezable ingredients can be blended with the cube portions right before serving.

Calorie Counting

Though most calorie counting is done by comparing spoon and cup measures of particular foods to a calorie chart, some families have found nutritional weight based dietary counters such as the 1450 Nutri-weigh Dietary Computer® helpful. This scale, and others like it, analyzes the nutritional content by portion size. It calculates calories, protein, carbohydrates, total sugars, fat, fiber from an extensive database.

Traveling with Homemade Blended Formulas

Some families will take all of their food preparation equipment with them and make complete meals while traveling. (The Vita-Mix blender sells a specially designed travel case for their blender.) Others prepare the food in advance and bring the food in proper storage containers. If the homemade blended formula is mixed ahead of time and taken on a trip, whether playgroup, picnic or day trip, it must be kept chilled.

Families must decide upon the equipment that works best for them. As always, transition slowly, carefully watching the child's response. Also move slowly with equipment purchases. It's not necessary to purchase all the fancy equipment and a big powerful blender at the beginning. There are many ways to try homemade blended formulas using commercial baby foods and easily blended cooked fruits and vegetables using an inexpensive blender and commonly available kitchen equipment. Once a family has seen that a homemade blended formula works for them and decides to move to a next level of preparation complexity, they can investigate the purchase of a more powerful blender.

For additional information on the Vita-Mix high powered blender and travel bag contact:
   Vita-Mix Corporation, Household Division, 8615 Usher Road, Cleveland, Ohio, 44138 USA
     www.vitamix.com/ Tel: 800-848-2649 FAX: 440-235-372

     Vita-Mix Corporation is pleased to offer a Medical Needs Discount Program, which is available to all eligible candidates. This discount program offers patients an opportunity to purchase a factory reconditioned machine at a significant discount. If you feel that you qualify for this discount, please contact Vita-Mix Corporation for details. Eligibility will be determined by Vita-Mix Corporation. Call 1-800-848-2649 or email household@vitamix.com for assistance and reference this code: ***07-0036-0011***.

For additional information on the Blendtec Total Blender Classic contact:
   Blendtec Corporate Headquarters, 1206 S. 1680 W. Orem Utah 84058
    www.blendtec.com Tel: 800-748-5400 FAX: 801-802-8584
   Blendtec offers a Medical Discount for eligible candidates. Call to inquire.

For additional information on the Nutri-weigh Dietary Computer® contact:
   Salter (the manufacturer) at http://www.salterhousewares.com

For more information on traveling with equipment see:
   Klein, M.D. and Morris, S.E. (2007). Chapter 22 – Traveling With Homemade Blended
   Formulas. *Homemade Blended Formula Handbook*. Tucson, AZ: Mealtime Notions, LLC

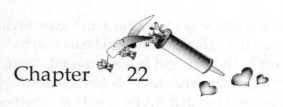

Traveling with Homemade Blended Formulas

Marsha Dunn Klein, M.Ed., OTR/L

Parents of tube fed children have discovered many creative ways to travel with homemade blended formulas. Many factors influence their mealtime decisions. These include length of the trip, types of foods chosen, and equipment required to prepare the food. Short playgroup excursions require different planning than a trip to a grandparent's house or a two-week vacation at a beach hotel.

Food Choices

Some families provide their tube fed child a diet of homemade blended purees at home, and they want to continue doing so when they travel. In preparing for the trip, they need to consider their specific needs for buying, preparing and storing the foods they'll be giving to their child.

For short trips, they may bring previously pre-pared blended meals, or meal components such as food ice cubes, and store them in an insulated pack, ice pack or on dry ice. For longer trips, some families pack their high-powered blender or send it ahead to their destination so they can provide the identical diet they prepare at home.

Many tube fed children eat a blended version of the same meals the whole family eats. At mealtimes they may be offered a plate of food to enjoy orally—tasting, nibbling and eating what they can—and then the remainder is blended at the end of the meal and provided in a bolus by tube. While traveling, it's relatively easy to do this with a home-cooked meal, or to order at a restaurant and take the leftovers back to the hotel for blending. Baby foods, vegetable and fruit juices, or dairy products can supplement the blended meals, as necessary.

Meal preparation for children who receive a combination of formula and commercial baby food also is similar to meal preparation at home.

Food and formula can be mixed by hand, although using a blender improves the consistency for tube feeding.

Families who provide only homemade foods to their tube fed children often choose to simplify while traveling and may change to a streamlined version of their blended diet. They may bring commercial formula and add extra baby foods to provide variation and calories. This may be easily managed using a regular blender that's easily available, allowing the family to leave their heavy-duty high-powered blender at home.

Still others choose to provide commercially available blended food meals such as Real Food Blends (www.realfoodblends.com) or food based formula such as Compleat® Pediatric so they can focus on the trip and not on food preparation. Check them out!

Orally fed children seem to do very well with travel variations in their diets: and so do most tube fed children.

Storage

Foods offered by tube need to be prepared and stored in safe and sanitary conditions. The usual recommendation is to defrost frozen homemade purees in the refrigerator. Many families put frozen purees in an insulated bag or ice chest with ice, ice packs, or dry ice. Homemade pureed foods always must be kept chilled to prevent bacterial growth and food spoilage. Canned formulas and commercial baby food store easily if they haven't been opened.

There are many excellent travel containers designed especially for keeping things cold, such as spouted liquid containers with tubular inserts that can be pre-frozen and screwed into the lid, remaining on the inside of the container. Many families have used these containers to store puree while out on short excursions. The spout can be easily popped open and puree squeezed directly into the syringe, creating a mess-free meal.

Mealtimes in Public

Parents have different comfort levels with the tube and tube feeding, and their emotions often surface when faced with feeding their children in public. Some families do all tube meals at home or in private, while others are comfortable using their usual tube feeding equipment in public restaurants and parks. It's a personal choice.

One Mother's Story

Bobby's mother took her whole family to the beach. She thought she was quite comfortable with the tube until she realized she'd forgotten 4-year-old Bobby's full-body (cover-up-the-button-tube) bathing suit. He wanted to swim with his siblings, so she was forced to let him swim in his underwear! Bobby's mother realized she WAS uncomfortable that everyone could see his feeding button and tube, but she decided that she was there for the day and he needed to be able to swim like the other children.

Of course, immediately another mother and five year old came by and with the great uninhibited innocence of childhood, the little girl pointed to the tube and asked, "What's that?" Bobby's Mom cringed at first and then formulated her answer.

"When Bobby was a baby, he didn't learn to eat like you did. This is a tube that he uses so he can eat." The little girl looked worried. "But, how does he eat strawberries?" Bobby's mother smiled and assured her that Bobby could eat strawberries, explaining that she blended them right up and put them into the tube. The little girl smiled a big smile and walked off happy that the little boy she had just met could have strawberries just like her. Even at the beach, Bobby could "eat" with the family!

Parent Thoughts

Many parents have offered suggestions about ways to comfortably travel with tube fed children and homemade blended formulas. One mother summarized her thoughts in the following way:

'Make it easy on yourself. When I first started traveling with my tube fed child, I would send entire suitcases of equipment ahead of time to the final destination. I would be exhausted during vacation trying to find the right foods and supplements, and finding the time to prepare all the blended foods in a different environment. Gradually I gave myself permission to cut corners, still providing good nutrition. Commercial formulas—though not what I like to provide my child as a steady diet— are well balanced, and by using them we could spend more vacation time 'vacationing' as a family. My orally fed children would have the occasional fast food meal. I began to see the commercial formula as the equivalent of a 'fast' meal with much more healthy food.`

For additional information on the Vita-Mix blender and travel bag contact:

Vita-Mix Corporation Household Division, 8615 Usher Road, Cleveland, OH 44128 USA
www.vitamin.com/

Vita-Mix Corporation is pleased to offer a Medical Needs Discount Program, which is available to all eligible candidates. This discount program offers patients an opportunity to purchase a factory reconditioned machine at a significant discount. If you feel that you qualify for this discount, please contact Vita-Mix Corporation for details. Eligibility will be determined by Vita-Mix Corporation. Call 1-800-848-2649 or email household@vitamix.com for assistance and reference this code: ***07-0036-0011***.

For additional information on the Blendtec Total Blender Classic contact:
Blendtec Corporate Headquarters, 1206 S. 1680 W. Orem Utah 84058
www.blendtec.com Tel: 800-748-5400 FAX: 801-802-8584

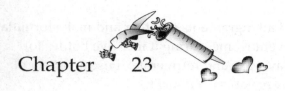

Chapter 23

A Parent's Perspective: A "No Frills" Approach

Frances Buoyer McDermott, M.S.,CCC-SLP

Initially, my knowledge of blenderized diets was purely professional. As a speech-language pathologist, I often recommended a variety of thickened liquid diets for my patients with swallowing disorders. I relied on the expertise of clinical dietitians to ensure they received adequate hydration and their nutritional requirements were met. Some thought me well prepared to take on the nutritional needs of my own son, who was born with significant disabilities. Thus began my journey in earnest into the world of formulas, feeding tubes and, eventually, blenderized diets.

During my son Thomas' first year of life, he was offered breast milk as well as a variety of formulas deemed appropriate for infants. He went through months of food allergy symptoms, gastro-esophageal reflux and projectile vomiting. After receiving a gastrostomy tube, Thomas still had severe retching and gagging. We began searching for new ways to make Thomas' feedings comfortable and pleasurable. We experimented with various delivery speeds and amounts in each meal. We explored comfortable positioning during tube feedings and relaxation through massage and music. Thomas' retching and gagging decreased, but he continued to cry and appeared uncomfortable. The next question mark was formula – what else could we try?

After Thomas' first birthday, we were told that he was now a toddler and had to have a "toddler formula." My question was, "What's a toddler formula?" The answer was "Pediasure® ." Though many families have good experiences with this formula, Thomas' retching and gagging had never been worse than when he was on it. After many desperate phone calls to the gastroenterologist and clinical dietitian, I saw an advertisement for Compleat® Pediatric – "a blenderized diet." It contained real, recognizable foods on the label, not the unrecognizable ingredients that are in so many commercial formulas.

We tried Compleat Pediatric for at least one month, but Thomas began having significant diarrhea. Our new dietitian discovered that the formula contained a great deal of apple juice, which didn't agree with Thomas. At this point I thought, why can't we just make our own formula? During my career I'd known several adult patients who blenderized foods at home and put them through their feeding tubes.

We had wonderful guidance from our clinical dietitian, who supported our interest in beginning a blenderized diet for Thomas. Thomas' blenderized diet recipe includes: soy milk, baby food jars of yellow vegetables, green vegetables, fruit and meat, flaxseed oil, baby oatmeal or rice cereal, and prune or pear juice.

Using commercially prepared baby foods in Thomas' blenderized formula has been a good choice for us. Organic baby foods are produced with strict guidelines and standards. The labeling is clear regarding food content (no additives or preservatives), calories and nutritional values such as protein, iron and calcium. It's easy to increase or reduce Thomas' calories or protein intake by a telephone consultation with his dietitian. We're clear on exactly what Thomas is eating and it's nutritional values.

As the mother of three children, the ease and convenience of a blenderized diet is important to me. Organic commercially prepared baby foods are readily available in supermarkets and local grocery stores. Other caregivers who feed Thomas know exactly what foods and what amounts to include in the blenderized formula. Measuring and cooking large amounts of food isn't necessary when using baby food purchased in the supermarket. I'm happy that I'm feeding Thomas healthy foods with as many choices as possible, and that it only takes me ten minutes each day to prepare his formula. It's a solution that works well for Thomas and for our family.

Additionally, our family has chosen to support Thomas' diet with glyconutritional and phytonutritional products from Mannatech® , as well as with a children's vitamin and other food-based supplements. Thomas has enjoyed increased wellness and health since we added these products to his diet. They're easy to add into the prepared formula. One batch of formula is divided into three tube feedings for one day. It's prepared in 10 to 15 minutes in a high-powered blender.

Thomas has enjoyed a blenderized diet for over six years now. He has progressed from having severe gastrointestinal discomfort and symptoms to essentially no symptoms.

Thomas enjoys helping select various fruits and vegetables; I offer him small tastes while he's making his choices. A blenderized diet allows for food selection and mealtime discussion. I like knowing what Thomas is eating every day, and I like being able to make food choices for him. He has the most well-rounded diet in our family!

Thomas' Blenderized Diet *

12 oz soy milk
6 tsp Ambrotose® (glyconutrient supplement)
4 Tbs. flaxseed oil
6 tsp PhytAloe® (phytonutrient supplement)
4 jars baby food meat
4 ImmunoSTART® tablets (immune support)
4 oz baby food green vegetable
3 Glyco.Bear® tablets (vitamin/mineral supplement)
4 oz baby food yellow vegetable
3 Sport tablets (phytosterol supplement)
4 oz (1 jar) baby food fruit
3 cc calcium carbonate
6 oz prune juice or pear juice
2 Tbsp Benefiber®
½ cup dry baby oatmeal or barley cereal

I blend all ingredients together and make formula each evening, measuring it into five bottles for next day's use and refrigerate. I use a variety of fruits, vegetables and meat.

Our total volume is approximately 36 oz or 1080 cc. This is divided into four feedings and is approximately 1,050 calories.

Thomas' Feeding Schedule
April 2006

Time	Formula	Water
6:00 AM	8 oz blenderized food diet – rinse tube with 2 oz water at the end of feeding	N/A
7:30 AM	8 oz blenderized food diet – rinse tube with 2 oz water at the end of feeding	
12:00 Noon		8 oz via G-tube
2:00 PM	12 oz blenderized food diet – rinse tube with 1 oz water at the end of feeding	N/A
6:00 PM	Food and/or thickened liquid by mouth	8 oz via G-tube
9:00 PM	16 oz or 480 cc blender-ized food diet – rinse tube with 1 oz water at the end of feeding	N/A

Thomas has multiple food allergies. Do not substitute foods or supplements without checking with your child's healthcare team.

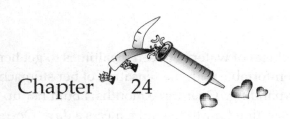

Chapter 24

A Parent's Perspective:
A "From Scratch" Approach

Lisa Larsen

At 14 months of age, a button type gastrostomy feeding tube was placed in my daughter Bella. On her doctor's recommendation, for more than two years she was fed a commercial formula. I was told that no supplemental water was required. During that time she became sickly and struggled to grow.

I enjoy preparing and eating food and I wanted to share that with my daughter. Also, in caring for my own health I actively sought nutritional and diet information and I wanted to use the same principles to support Bella's health. I already knew what her health was like on the commercial formula and I wanted to see if she could improve with dietary changes that included whole foods and supplemental water. I had no idea where to start, so I contacted her pediatrician and dietitian. Both said they had no experience with this type of food transition. They assured me the commercial formula provided all she needed. I was left to figure it out for myself.

In order to avoid a possible allergic reaction to any food, I transitioned Bella off the commercial formula very slowly and carefully. I knew I wanted a diet that was low-allergen and easily digestible. As she gradually transitioned to the initial blended diet, her health improved. As her health improved I became more comfortable and tried lots of variations. As I put the mixture in her tube, I would imagine a plate of rice, chicken and vegetables that she was eating and enjoying! What a difference our homemade blended formula made for both of us!

Making the Change

Where did I start? I read a lot about food allergies before transitioning Bella off the commercial formula. One point that was stressed in books was that the body becomes habituated to a food when it is given daily, even if the body is allergic

to it. In order to safely remove the food from the diet with the least stress on the body, it must be done slowly, or risk throwing the body into a health crisis.

Since Bella already was sickly, I dared not risk taxing her system any more. I decided to approach the transition period in the same manner that's recommended for introducing foods to babies – one food at a time for four to seven days. This method allowed me to "clear" each individual food, so if I got a negative reaction from Bella, I knew which food or herb was causing the problem.

I began by adding small amounts of a low-allergen nutritional supplement, Ultracare for Kids® by Metagenics®, to her formula. I did this for about a month, gradually increasing the supplement and decreasing some of the formula, calorie for calorie. Though the commercial formula was still her "base," there was less of it. Next, I began adding a little chicken broth made with chicken, carrots and celery. I did this for two weeks.

Knowing she was stable and tolerating the supplement and broth, I started adding solid foods. I began with a week of organic baby food carrots—a little bit the first day and an increasing quantity each day. This process continued with other vegetables. Once I cleared a vegetable, I would quit using it and try the next vegetable. I continued using broth and the supplement daily, even though the vegetable changed each week. With every change in her diet, we carefully monitored her growth and her health.

Once we cleared seven vegetables, I started introducing congee. Congee is an easily digested, slow-cooked porridge that's a staple of the diet in many Asian countries. I tried brown rice first, because it's the main ingredient in the supplement we chose. Next I tried millet, then quinoa, oatmeal and amaranth. Bella didn't tolerate the amaranth at all and the quinoa was "so-so". Thus I knew to stick with rice, millet and oatmeal.

Finally I introduced chicken. I figured her body would tolerate chicken since she had been receiving chicken broth for some time. Interestingly, once I introduced chicken through her tube, my highly "non-oral" child started eating chicken by mouth! Then she started reaching for the same grains and vegetables she was receiving through her tube.

Over time, I began adding different meats, but the limiting factor was the blender we were using. Because my personal preference was to prepare my own meats rather than use baby food meats, I needed to invest in a good high-powered blender. A nurse told me about the Vita-Mix high powered blender. It so completely pureed all foods that I no longer needed to worry about clogging the tube, and our food options expanded. This blender allowed me to blend any kind of meat, eliminating the stringiness that my household blender couldn't remove. I discovered creative ways to slow cook the meats in different broths. As I got comfort-able, I added various well-researched herbs and spices to the broth base.

The last nutritional component I cleared with Bella was oil. Oils are harder to digest, so I gave her body plenty of time to get accustomed to pro-cessing other foods before introducing oils. I began with flax oil, starting with small quantities and building to larger amounts. Next came olive oil, and occasionally canola or sesame oil— although I've read such great things about olive oil that I didn't worry about using it every day.

By this point, the feeding pump was no longer an option. The homemade mixture was so thick I needed to use a syringe with a plunger. I would use 60 ml (cc) syringes to slowly put the food in her tummy. Since her body had been used to the slow drip of a pump (i.e., hour-long feedings), I needed to build her tolerance for quantity. I used boluses of water between mealtimes to get her comfortable with the sensation of her stomach expanding. Over three months, I built her up to tolerating four to five tube meals a day. Once I eliminated the commercial formula completely and increased her water intake, she was able to tolerate four fairly large feedings a day, with water in between. Her volume tolerance was important for ensuring she received sufficient calories for growth, without having to rely on the concen-trated calories in the commercial formula.

Finally in September 1997, it was time to eliminate the commercial formula for good. Even though I had carefully cleared the foods and believed that the whole-food purees were meeting her needs, I'd grown accustom to the convenience of the commercial formula and the security it offered calorically. I knew how many calories were in every can and how many cans a day my child needed to grow. Switching to a new diet meant I was letting go of that information.

I had worked with three dietitians by this time and all of them wanted me to add soy or dairy as a primary food source. Although Bella's diet occasionally included soy milk, I wasn't comfort-able making soy or dairy the primary food source because they're known allergens for many people. I didn't want to risk it. Bella was doing well with all the new foods and starting to thrive. Instinctively, I knew our whole-food diet was working without soy or dairy as its base. So I told myself that mothers had been feeding their children effectively since the beginning of time and that I could do that too. I had to make peace with the fact that I was going against expert advice. My child's growth and health definitely were improving and I had my pediatrician's support. I had to find that place that exists inside all primary caregivers who know what's best for their child.

I remember opening the last can of commercial formula that I ever used and pouring it into my nourishing mixture of broth, oil, meat, grains and vegetables. By this point I was using only one can a day, but it was still a known calorie source.

I was afraid and excited all at once. The next day I gave Bella a whole day of whole foods. Even though I had no idea about the calories, I imagined each tube feeding as a plate of food. For the first time the tube became a friend because I now was able to feed my child a "perfect diet".... one that included foods that most of her peers refused to eat!

Bella Today

In December 2002, my sister was caring for Bella while I was out of town. They ran out of tube mixture. By this point, Bella was getting minimal tube food and was eating well by mouth. Because my sister didn't know how to make the tube food, she told Bella she would have to eat everything with her mouth. Bella agreed. By the time I got home, Bella had been self sustaining for four days. Once she saw me, she cried for the tube. However, with my husband's support, I was able to resist her complaints and encourage her to keep eating by mouth. On several occasions, my husband spent an hour sitting at the dinner table with Bella because she wanted tube food not mouth food. He would encourage her and wait for her to decide to eat by mouth. With time and patience, the cycle changed.

In May of 2003, her site was surgically sealed. Now she has a faint little scar on her tummy that she proudly shows doctors, therapists and tube fed children and their parents.

Today Bella is nearly 13 years old and in middle school. Since becoming an oral eater, she jumped from the fourth percentile for weight to the 25th. Her doctor was amazed by her sudden increase. She eats three meals a day and several snacks. She LOVES food. She loves to eat and cook, and she eats a huge variety: soy products, salads, pastas, goat cheese, pizza, fruit, mashed potatoes. Her favorite restaurant is a local buffet. She relishes the variety of foods offered and enjoys picking them herself. After a salad and main dish, she always cruises the dessert bar.

I still watch Bella eat with joy and awe. I vividly remember the ten years of tube feeding and all the cooking and blending I did. It was relentless. I remember the times I felt overwhelmed and exhausted. Then I look across the table to see her scraping her ice cream bowl, not wanting to miss a drop, and I'm grateful. I am grateful Bella grew up smelling wonderful, healthy food being cooked just for her. I am grateful the tube kept her well fed until she could feed herself. I am especially grateful I trusted my inner voice, which said I could feed my daughter real, home-cooked food through her tube.

Bella's Homemade Blended Formula Recipes

Bella's recipes were nutritionally analyzed by a dietitian, on the recommendation of her feeding therapist. The dietitian was pleased with the nutritional variation the recipes provided. We all learned from the journey. Bella thrived and felt great. Her pediatrician and dietitian now have more information about how to help the next parent who asks, and we all learned to work together to change the life of my child.

Bella's Basic Recipe

½ jar of Bella's congee
⅓ jar of broth
⅓ - ½ jar meat
4 scoops of Ultracare for Kids®
5 capsules of Jarrow® acidophilus with FOS
    (I opened the capsules and pour contents in
    the blender, but they can be purchased in
    powdered form)
2-4 Tbsp flax oil
2-4 Tbsp oil
    (We rotated between extra virgin olive,
    canola and sesame oils.)
5-6 jars of green vegetables
    (Select peas, green beans, spinach or
    summer vegetable mix)
1-2 jars of an orange vegetable
    (Select carrots, winter squash or sweet potato)

All of the individual fresh ingredients are processed ahead of time with the high powered blender and stored in the refrigerator in glass jars. When each meal is prepared these separate ingredients are blended together at a low variable speed of the Vita-Mix high powered blender or with a regular blender to make a smooth mixture that will pass easily through the feeding tube.

In the past we steamed fresh or frozen vegetables and blended them in the high powered blender. However, to save time, we transitioned into using baby food in four-ounce jars.

Bella's basic recipe was frequently modified by the addition of some of the following options: liquid vitamins, honey, maple syrup, molasses, pureed fruits, scrambled eggs, well-cooked beans, yogurt, spirulina, seaweed, bee pollen, protein powder, roasted almond butter, soy milk and rice milk.

Chicken Broth

2 cups sliced organic fresh ginger
   (for stomach health)
2-3 pounds of carrots (washed and cut up)
Fresh rosemary and thyme (2 bunches each)
2 whole organic chickens with innards discarded
   (Wash. Smell chickens when purchasing.
    Fresh chickens should have NO odor.)
1 bunch of celery (washed and chopped)
1 tsp sea salt
2-3 gallons of filtered water

Bring the mixture to a boil and skim off the foam. Cook on the lowest temperature possible that allows for a slow rolling boil. Cover. Cook for 6-7 hours. Strain and press through a strainer of cheesecloth. Use a wide funnel and put the broth in clean jars. Put on a two-piece canning lid. Cool to room temperature and refrigerate.

Be sure each of these ingredients works well for your child before adding them to the broth.

Congee

Combine 5 cups of filtered water and 1 cup of well-washed grain. Add favorite herbs and a pinch of sea salt (optional). Cover. Cook on low in a crock pot for 8 hours. Let cool a bit and pour into your blender. Blend well and store in Mason jars with lid in the refrigerator.

Bella's preferred grains: Organic short-grain brown rice, millet and oatmeal

Bella's preferred spices: Nutmeg, cloves, allspice, cinnamon, ginger

Meat Mixture

Bella gets either boneless, skinless chicken breasts or turkey tenders because dark meat didn't agree with her. With the help of the high powered blender, she has successfully gotten steak, lamb and fish (which doesn't need as long to cook).

   3-4 pounds of meat in a large crockpot
   2-3 cups of filtered water and herbs

Put meat, herbs and water into the pot and cover. Cook on low for about 8 hours or high for about 5 hours. Experiment because the altitude, brand of cooking pot, type and quantity of meat can change the cooking time. You want the meat to be well cooked so that it flakes easily. Let it cool a bit.

Place ¼ of the meat and liquid into the high powered blender and blenderize until smooth. Add more of the liquid as needed. Pour into wide mouth glass jars and put the lid on. Repeat the process until all the meat is blenderized and in jars. Use plain filtered water if you run out of liquid in the crock pot.

Bella's preferred herbs: Sea salt, sage, marjoram, rosemary, thyme, ginger, powdered garlic, powdered onion. (Clear each herb one at a time before adding them to the mixture.)

Yummy Breakfast Combination

Combine congee, filtered water, honey, maple syrup or molasses, banana and blueberries. Blend well. Strawberries, raspberries and blackberries all have big seeds that got stuck in Bella's tube, so they were avoided.

Bella's Recipes for Gastrointestinal Support

Bella has had a long history of reflux and general gastrointestinal discomfort. We've found a number of teas that support her digestion and comfort when she's having difficulty.

Chamomile Tea

Cover 2 heaping tablespoons of chamomile with 1½ cups of boiling filtered water. Cover and let steep about 20 minutes until a deep golden color. It is bitter to the taste. Bella gets 2 ounces at a time, usually prior to a meal, for tummy support. I use a diluted version first. The chamomile plant is a member of the ragweed family, so I knew if a child is allergic to ragweed, not to use chamomile.

Rosemary Tea

Combine 2 cups of filtered water and 1 teaspoon of dried rosemary in a covered pan and simmer, boil for 20 minutes. This tea can be offered warm or cool. I personally take this occasionally for tummy upset. Only use occasionally. Try a diluted version first.

Fresh Ginger Tea

Peel and slice organic fresh ginger root and simmer-boil covered in filtered water for 20-30 minutes. The amount of ginger depends on your taste. It should be strong but drinkable. It can be offered with honey for older children. It's nice for the whole family. Only use a diluted version first.

This has been Bella's story. The foods and supplements chosen and the approach taken are personal and specific to Bella's family. Check with your child's physician before embarking on any dietary changes.

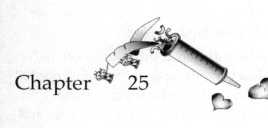

Anatomy of a Recipe

Suzanne Evans Morris, Ph.D., Jude Trautlein, R.D.,
Ellen Duperret, R.D.,
Marsha Dunn Klein, M.Ed., OTR/L

Chapter 25

The first question many parents and professionals ask when beginning to use a homemade blended formula is "What recipe should I use for my child?" This is fueled by a belief that there's a "best" recipe that provides the caloric and nutrient needs for their youngster.

When parents consult other parents to learn what they're including in their homemade blended formulas, they often find that formulas designed for other children don't fit the specific needs of their own child.

It takes different recipes to feed children who are older or younger, more or less active, more or less food-sensitive, and who require more or less volume, calories or fluid.

Parents quickly realize that the "best" recipe for homemade blended formulas doesn't exist. Additionally, they often discover that a dietary plan recommended by a dietitian who hasn't worked with homemade blended formulas may not blend well, or may result in such a large amount of food that their child can't handle the volume.

Ultimately, parents do the very best they can, based on what they know about foods and nutrition. But they often feel frustrated, or discover that their child isn't growing well on the new formula. Some will ultimately give up the new venture and go back to commercial formulas.

Clearly, success in creating a well-balanced home-made blended formula for each unique child takes planning, information and support. A good place to start is learning the complementary parts, or "anatomy" of any recipe.

The Anatomy of a Recipe

Initially, we had planned to create a small collection of recipes with examples of many different formulas for children with different growth and health needs. This is what parents are asking for, and it seemed a reasonable idea. However, as we explored this further, we realized this concept didn't fit with our evolving knowledge and philosophy. There are a wide variety of nutritional considerations in planning a diet for any child or adult. Our major goal is to give parents and professionals a set of tools and strategies for developing an individualized program that works best for their unique children.

Our philosophy is that menu planning for a tube fed child should follow the same basic food choice guidelines as for an orally fed child with similar growth and health needs. Parents would not ask for a single recipe or menu for an orally fed child, so why would this limited concept be appropriate for a tube fed child whose food is blended into a formula instead of offered on a plate?

The concept of looking at the anatomy of a recipe makes a great deal of sense because it offers parents and professionals the tools for designing their own recipes, instead of just selecting a pre-designed recipe that has the "best fit."

We speak of "anatomy" because the anatomy of the human body suggests a collection of different parts that are connected to each other in specific ways that support each other. For example, the jaw, tongue, lips and cheeks are all parts of the anatomy of the mouth. Each part is related intimately to the other parts. The jaw provides the stability that enables the lips and tongue to move with greater independence. The tongue, jaw and lips work together with exquisite timing and coordination when we eat and drink. If there's too much or too little involvement of one part, the whole process of sucking, swallowing or chewing is affected.

The same concept applies to the anatomy of a recipe. Carbohydrates, proteins, fats and calories form the skeletal structure of the recipe; vitamins, minerals, phytonutrients and fiber make up other parts. Food groups, food equivalents, diversity and personal food preferences all are parts. When there's too much or too little of one of these parts, the anatomy is out of balance and nutrition for growth and health is compromised.

While recipe anatomy follows a basic structure, every recipe or menu depends on a set of characteristics defined by the child. These include:

The Child's Age

Infants need a larger number of calories per pound than toddlers because they grow very rapidly during the first 6-12 months. Although toddlers and preschoolers have a slower rate of growth, they eat a larger number of calories because their body weight is greater. During growth spurts, most children have larger appetites and take in more calories.

The Child's Height and Weight

These measurements also help determine the appropriate number of calories and nutrients. Taller or heavier children require more calories to maintain their current rate of growth.

The Child's Personal Patterns of Growth

Each child's personal growth pattern can be represented by a series of connected points on a growth chart. Some children have a consistent growth curve at the 50th percentile level, while others are at the 25th percentile. Still others may remain in the 5th percentile throughout infancy and early childhood. Each of these patterns can be normal for a given child.

The Child's Activity Level

Children vary greatly in their activity level throughout the day. Very active children burn up a large number of calories; sedentary children don't use many calories. The greater the activity level, the higher the number of calories the child needs each day.

The Child's Special Medical Needs

A child's medical diagnosis influences both his or her activity level and the specific nutrients needed each day. For example, a child with spastic cerebral palsy typically has very stiff muscles and very little spontaneous movement or activity, therefore requiring fewer calories per pound. But a child with athetoid cerebral palsy has muscles that are constantly contracting and relaxing as muscle tone fluctuates. This burns up many calories, even though the child may be unable to walk or run.

In addition, medications may change dietary needs. For example, anticonvulsants for seizures, or acid-reducing medications for reflux can cause poor absorption of some vitamins and minerals. These children may need higher levels of these nutrients in their diet.

The Child's Allergies, Food Intolerances or Special Dietary Restrictions

Foods that cause problems should be eliminated from the diet or eaten infrequently. Other foods should be substituted that provide the same nutrients. Some children have dietary restrictions based on metabolic needs or family preferences. Honoring these needs influences the specific foods included in a homemade blended formula.

The Foods Easily Accepted by the Body

Prior to serving homemade foods, the general recommendation is to introduce each food one at a time to be sure the child's body accepts it easily. Once the child demonstrates the ability to handle a variety of foods, these foods can be blended together in healthful combinations.

Designing a Menu for Children

Parents feed their children according to formal and informal guidelines for calories and nutrients. In most families, adults select foods for the meal, which determines the nutrients and calories available to the child. Ideally, the child's appetite and familiarity with different foods will determine the level of nutrients and calories eaten at each meal.

Unfortunately, the dietary choices offered to orally fed children often are determined by advertising, a fast food culture and parental convenience. As a result, a growing proportion of children are becoming overweight and obese due to eating more calories than are needed by their bodies. Inadequate nutrient levels also are reflected in the increase in chronic diseases such as Type II diabetes and asthma. Many professionals also ascribe the increase in attention deficit disorders and learning disabilities to dietary problems.

ChooseMyPlate

Pediatricians and dietitians provide guidance to parents based on a number of nutritional guidelines. The most common set of recommendations comes from the ChooseMyPlate guidelines developed by the U.S. Department of Agriculture (USDA). The USDA's ChooseMyPlate was published in 2011.

ChooseMyPlate nutrition messaging is based on the 2010 Dietary Guidelines for American's two years old and older. MyPlate illustrates five food groups that are the building blocks for a healthy diet. The ChooseMyPlate and its SuperTracker program provide tools to learn about healthy eating and manage weight and calorie intake. The SuperTracker helps track what a person eats and drinks and provides a personalized diet and activity plan. It supports physical activity as a part of daily health and nutrition.

In ChooseMyPlate, the calorie needs of each person are calculated based on age, gender and activity level. This information is translated into the measured amounts of grain, vegetables, fruits, meat and beans, dairy and oils.

With children, it's important to remember that this is only a guideline and not a fixed dietary plan that specifies the exact intake that a child must consume each day. The variations within the structured guidelines of ChooseMyPlate allow for wide variation that supports dietary diversity.

Role and Use of Recipes

Once parents have a general set of guidelines for feeding their children, they can create specific meals in a variety of different ways.

Some families develop a fixed set of meal patterns and don't vary from them. Monday nights are fried chicken, mashed potatoes and peas; Tuesday nights are macaroni and cheese with green beans; Wednesdays are spaghetti and meatballs with a green salad.

Some families buy frozen prepared foods or purchase carryout meals from a local restaurant, to accommodate their specific time constraints and interest in meal preparation. Others cook from recipes, which they may adapt to their family's taste preferences. No matter the preparation method, with time and experience, family chefs create mealtime menus based on these guiding questions: What's in a healthy diet? What food groups would I like to offer at each meal? How much of each food is appropriate for my child?

When families begin to make their own meals rather than purchasing prepared foods, they're often drawn to recipe books. These offer a wonderful way to increase interest in new foods and expand mealtime variety. Recipe books also increase the confidence of the cook and encourage trying something new with a greater guarantee of "success."

Let's look at an example of a recipe modification that expands mealtime experiences within the family. Spaghetti with tomato sauce is a popular dinner choice. The most common version consists primarily of spaghetti pasta with a smooth sauce based on tomatoes, herbs and cheese. Parents may prepare the sauce from scratch or use a commercially prepared sauce from a jar. Adding a variety of vegetables to the sauce modifies the recipe, as does hamburger, sausage or tofu. Different herbs and spices create different tastes. Different preparation styles create different textures. Spaghetti recipe variations are infinite.

Designing a Formula Menu for Tube Fed Children

Designing a homemade blended formula menu for the tube fed child uses the same basic pattern as is used for an orally fed child -- with a few differences. Parents find that some foods blend well together while others do not. In most instances, compatible foods are discovered by trial and error, since much depends on the way the food is cooked and the type of blender used to blend it up.

Because food must be mixed with liquid to make it thin enough to pass through a feeding tube, the final volume of formula can pose a problem for some children. Typically, children can handle a larger volume of homemade blended formula than the thinner commercial formula. However, some continue to need a formula that provides needed calories and nutrients in as small a serving as possible. Dietitians use the terms "caloric density" and "nutrient density" to describe foods that pack a large number of calories or nutrients into a relatively small volume.

Figuring Out the Dietary Needs of a Specific Child

Using mathematical formulas and charts, dietitians make the best educated guess about the correct number of calories per ounce of formula and the total volume of formula needed each day for a specific child. These calculations are based on averages for the child's age, height, weight and activity level (as detailed above).

This recommendation becomes a guideline or a starting point. The proof of the correctness of the initial recommendation is the child's continued healthy growth. Calories will be increased or decreased depending on growth and health.

Theme and Variation

Successful recipes are built on a central theme of nutritional and caloric components. The amount of each of the components is specified, but the variations create dietary diversity that supports the child's nutritional needs.

Fruits change   Vegetables change
Grains change   Proteins change
Oils and fats change

The Core Guidelines

Our simple method for planning a child's homemade blended formula starts with the number of calories the child currently is receiving through the tube, and builds through food choices based on the USDA ChooseMyPlate planning suggestions. Inherent in this system is parental choice and food variation. These guidelines provide the tools that allow parents to decide on a few favorite recipes, and then vary them every day or week to be unique. Food ingredients can be commercially prepared, fresh, or from frozen homemade ice cubes made in advance. Individual meals can be created for breakfast, lunch and dinner, or foods can be blended all together into one formula that's served throughout the day.

Using these guidelines and a healthy dose of trial-and-error, parents ultimately will discover the "best" personalized homemade blended formula for their special child's needs.

For more information on core guidelines for homemade blended formulas, see:

Klein, M.D. and Morris, S.E. (2007). Chapter 26 – Core Guidelines for a Homemade Blended Formula. *Homemade Blended Formula Handbook*. TucsonAZ: Mealtime Notions, LLC.

For additional information about the ChooseMyPlate see:

ChooseMyPlate at www.choosemyplate.gov

For more information on expanding homemade blended formulas with recipes, see:

Karamel, A. (2004). *First Meals*. New York, NY: DK Publishing.

Karamel, A. (2006). *Top 100 Baby Purees: 100 Quick and Easy Meals for a Healthy and Happy Baby*.

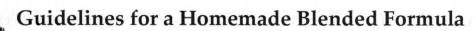

Guidelines for a Homemade Blended Formula

Chapter 26   Jude Trautlein, R.D., Ellen Duperret, R.D.,
Marsha Dunn Klein, M.Ed., OTR/L,
Suzanne Evans Morris, Ph.D, CCC

If you're reading this chapter, you've:

- made a decision to gradually introduce a form of homemade blended formula to your child;

- gained an overall sense of the importance of moving slowly and deliberately to identify the most appropriate combination of foods to include; and

- know that the technique and environment in which the formula is offered to the child is just as important as the food and liquid content.

Now you're ready to work with core guideline concepts to create and fine-tune a series of personalized recipes that will meet your child's nutritional needs as he or she transitions from a commercial formula or breastmilk to a homemade blended formula.

Initial Preparation

Check with your child's physician and dietitian to see if a homemade blended formula is right for your child. Determine special dietary restrictions or considerations.

Ensure your child's digestive system comfortably accepts a number of different foods, and that these foods are introduced one at a time, with a period of observation of the child's response to each.

Initially, these foods are presented as additions to commercial formula or breast milk infant diets. Once your child's system accepts or tolerates a variety of different foods from each food group, you may consider offering combinations of foods together in bolus meals. Gradually the bolus meal calories can take the place of commercial formula as your child comfortably tolerates the volume needed for daily nutritional needs.

A *Homemade Blended Formula Tolerance Chart* is provided on page 115 for tracking a child's four day response to new foods or combinations of foods. As you can see from the chart, familiar foods, new foods, bowel movements, vomiting and gagging episodes, discomfort responses and rashes or mucus changes can be charted. This will allow you to monitor your child's responses and create your own lists of foods and food combinations.

Sample Section of Daily Calorie Guidelines Chart

	Male				Female		
Age	**Sedentary**	**Moderately Active**	**Active**	**Age**	**Sedentary**	**Moderately Active**	**Active**
2 yrs	1000	1000	1000	2 years	1000	1000	1000
3 yrs	1000	1400	1400	3 years	1000	1200	1400
4 yrs	1200	1400	1600	4 years	1200	1400	1400
5 yrs	1200	1400	1600	5 years	1200	1400	1600
6 yrs	1400	1600	1800	6 years	1200	1400	1600

Based on My Pyramid Food Intake Pattern Calorie Levels for growth, April 2005   (www.mypyramid.gov)

Complete chart can be found at end of this chapter.

Calorie Goal

An estimated *Calorie Goal* is a starting point for diet calculations. Use current number of calories your child is receiving by tube each day OR estimate the number of calories based on your child's age, gender and activity level using the *Daily Calorie Guidelines* which are located in entirety at the end of this chapter (sample section previous page) OR ask your child's dietitian for help. *Daily Calorie Guidelines* are based on the US Department of Agriculture (USDA) guidelines for growth.

Children grow appropriately when they receive adequate nutrition, including calories and a variety of other of nutrients. Remember this is a starting point, a guideline only. Your child may need more or less calories for proper growth. The calorie goal recommendation can be modified up or down, based on how well the child grows and the child's overall level of health.

For example, the starting point for a child who receives five containers of Pediasure® per day would be the calories per container (237) times 5, for a total of 1185 calories per day. As another example, on the *Daily Calorie Guidelines Chart*, a 6-year-old boy who is sedentary may need approximately 1400 calories per day, whereas an active 6-year-old girl may need 1600 calories per day. When an estimated calorie level is used, the child's growth must be monitored to ensure appropriate growth.

Homemade Blended Formula Worksheets

A series of *Homemade Blended Formula Worksheets* (sample below) are included at the end of this chapter for the target number of calories you have selected. There are specific *Homemade Blended Formula Worksheets* available for calorie goals of 1000 to 3200 calories, in 200-calorie increments.

Selecting Foods for the Homemade Blended Formula

Using the worksheet for the specific calorie level, choose foods in amounts recommended from each of the food groups. Recommendations are based on the USDA MyPyramid and ChooseMyPlate food guidance system developed in 2005 and then in 2011. The ChooseMyPlate provides a visual guideline for healthy nutrition.

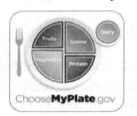

Visit the Web site (www.choosemyplate.gov) for additional information.

Sample Homemade Blended Formula Worksheet
1000 Calories

Food Group	Tip	Goal: Based on a 1000 Calorie Pattern	List Foods Chosen	Calories
GRAINS	Make at least half your grains whole grains	**3 one-ounce equivalents** (A one-ounce equivalent is about 1 slice of bread, or 1 cup dry cereal, or ½ cup cooked rice, pasta or cereal)		
VEGETABLES	Choose vegetables of different colors for dietary diversity	**1 cup**		
FRUITS	Consider fruits for most choices rather than juices and choose a variety of colors for dietary diversity	**1 cup**		
MILK/MILK SUBSTITUTES	Milks and yogurts tend to blend more easily than cheese	**2 cups**		
MEATS, BEANS, NUTS	Vary choices among meats, poultry, fish, legumes, nuts and seeds	**2 one-ounce equivalents** (A one-ounce equivalent is 1 ounce meat, poultry or fish; 1 egg, 1 tablespoon peanut butter; ½ ounce nuts; or ¼ cup cooked legumes)		
FATS	Choose olive, canola, flax for better health	**3 teaspoons**		
			Subtotal Calories:	
EXTRAS	For children under age 2, add additional fats for brain development. For older children, calories can come from any source.		**Total Extra Calories:**	
			Total Calories:	

Adhering to these guidelines will provide the minimum basic essential nutrient needs of the child, if a variety of different foods within each food group are chosen. There will be some fluctuation in the daily calorie levels based on the foods chosen -- bananas have more calories than peaches, and carrots have more calories than green beans.

Using a calorie reference chart, calculate the total number of calories in the foods you have chosen. If the total is less than the *Calorie Goal* for the day as in the recommended equivalents, add additional food to meet the daily calorie requirements. For children under the age of two, add additional fats for brain development. For other children, calories can come from any source.

Comparison of Food Recommendations for 1000– and 2000-Calorie Pattern

Food Group	1000-Calorie Pattern	2000-Calorie Pattern
Grains	3 one-ounce equivalents	6 one-ounce equivalents
Vegetables	1 cup	2.5 cups
Fruits	1 cup	2 cups
Milk/ Milk Substitute	2 cups	3 cups
Meat, Beans, Nuts	2 one-ounce equivalents	5 one-ounce equivalents
Fats	3 teaspoons	6 teaspoons

Adapted from MyPyramid worksheet, www.MyPyramid.gov. Food recommendations based on USDA dietary guidelines for Americans, 2005, and the Food Pyramid.

Example of the Core System

For example, imagine a little girl named Jenny who needs about 1000 calories per day to grow. The concepts in MyPyramid, or ChooseMyPlate with the sample formula worksheet for 1000 calories, we can observe how her homemade blended diet evolves.

Sample of Homemade Blended Formula Worksheet for "Jenny" Day One

Food Group	Tip	Goal: Based on a 1000 Calorie Pattern	Choices *for Jenny*	Calories
GRAINS	Make at least half your grains whole grains	3 one-ounce equivalents (A one-ounce equivalent is about 1 slice of bread, or 1 cup dry cereal, or ½ cup cooked rice, pasta or cereal)	1 cup instant Cream of Wheat (prepared) 1/2 cup dry oatmeal (cooked)	154 150
VEGETABLES	Choose vegetables of different colors for dietary diversity	1 cup	1/2 cup canned sweet potato 1/2 cup broccoli	91 15
FRUITS	Consider fruits for most choices rather than juices; choose a variety of colors for dietary diversity	1 cup	1/2 cup blue-berries 1/2 banana	35 50
MILK OR MILK SUBSTITUTE	Milks and yogurts tend to blend more easily than cheese	2 cups	1 cup whole milk 1 cup plain yogurt	150 150
MEATS, BEANS, NUTS	Vary choices among meats, poultry, fish, legumes, nuts and seeds	2 one-ounce equivalents (A one-ounce equivalent is 1 ounce meat, poultry or fish; 1 egg, 1 tablespoon peanut butter; ½ ounce nuts; or ¼ cup cooked legumes)	2 ounces cooked ground beef	142
FATS	Choose olive, canola, flax for better health	3 teaspoons	3 teaspoons olive oil	120
			Subtotal	1057

Comments Day One: Good job! The calorie level is close enough to 1000. Let's look at the next example.

Sample of Homemade Blended Formula Worksheet for "Jenny" Day Two

Food Group	Tip	Goal: Based on a 1000 Calorie Pattern	Choices *for Jenny*	Calories
GRAINS	Make at least half your grains whole grains	3 one-ounce equivalents (A one-ounce equivalent is about 1 slice of bread, or 1 cup dry cereal, or ½ cup cooked rice, pasta or cereal)	*1 cup brown rice*	216
			1/2 cup barley	97
VEGETABLES	Choose vegetables of different colors for dietary diversity	1 cup	*1/2 cup corn*	76
			1/2 cup parsnips	63
FRUITS	Consider fruits for most choices rather than juices;choose a variety of colors for dietary diversity	1 cup	*1/2 cup papaya*	27
			1/2 cup grapes	30
MILK OR MILK SUBSTITUTE	Milks and yogurts tend to blend more easily than cheese	2 cups	*2 cup soy milk*	200
MEATS, BEANS, NUTS	Vary choices among meats, poultry, fish, legumes, nuts and seeds	2 one-ounce equivalents (A one-ounce equivalent is 1 ounce meat, poultry or fish; 1 egg, 1 table-spoon peanut butter; ½ ounce nuts; or ¼ cup cooked legumes)	*1/2 cup garbanzos*	135
FATS	Choose olive, canola, flax for better health	3 teaspoons	*3 teaspoons canola oil*	120
			Subtotal	964

Comments Day Two: Good job! The calorie level is close enough! Averaging the calorie subtotals for day one and day two equals about 1000 calories.

Sample of Homemade Blended Formula Worksheet for "Jenny" Day Three

Food Group	Tip	Goal: Based on a 1000 Calorie Pattern	Choices *for Jenny*	Calories
GRAINS	Make at least half your grains whole grains	3 one-ounce equivalents (A one-ounce equivalent is about 1 slice of bread, or 1 cup dry cereal, or ½ cup cooked rice, pasta or cereal)	*1 cup oatmeal*	148
			1/2 cup wild rice	82
VEGETABLES	Choose vegetables of different colors for dietary diversity	1 cup	*1/2 cup asparagus*	22
			1/2 cup boiled cabbage	17
FRUITS	Consider fruits for most choices rather than juices;choose a variety of colors for dietary diversity	1 cup	*1/2 unsweetened apple sauce*	52
			1/2 cup peaches, canned in juice	54
MILK OR MILK SUBSTITUTE	Milks and yogurts tend to blend more easily than cheese	2 cups	*2 cups soy milk*	200
MEATS, BEANS, NUTS	Vary choices among meats, poultry, fish, legumes, nuts and seeds	2 one-ounce equivalents (A one-ounce equivalent is 1 ounce meat, poultry or fish; 1 egg, 1 table-spoon peanut butter; ½ ounce nuts; or ¼ cup cooked legumes)	*1 ounce chicken breast*	47
			1 ounce cod fish	30
FATS	Choose olive, canola, flax for better health	3 teaspoons	*3 teaspoons flax seed oil*	120
			Subtotal	772

Comments for Day Three:
On day three, the total was NOT close enough to 1000 with the specific foods chosen.
Her family needed to add more calories. Shown are the extras they chose to add.

Food Group	Tip	Goal: Based on a 1000 Calorie Pattern	Choices *for Jenny*	Calories
EXTRAS	For children under age 2, add additional fats for brain development. For older children, calories can come from any source.	Add about 228 calories.	*1/2 avocado* *1 tablespoon black strap molasses* *1 ounce prune juice*	*160* *47* *23*
			Subtotal of extras New Total Daily Calories	*230* *1002*

Creating the Daily Homemade Blended Formula

- Blend all the ingredients to proper consistency. (Extra water may need to be added.)
- Measure the total blended volume in ounces (oz) or milliliters (ml/cc).
- Divide the calorie total by the volume (in ounces or milliliters) to determine the calories per ounce or calories per milliliters. (For example, if Jenny's sample day three volume totaled 33 ounces, her formula would be 1002 calories divided by 33 ounces, which would equal 30 calories per ounce.)
- Present each new food individually and carefully observe the child's reaction. Chart these observations on the *Homemade Blended Formula Tolerance Chart* at the end of this chapter.
- Monitor your child's growth and weight with regular health checks.

For additional information on creating a homemade blended formula see:

Klein, M.D. and Morris, S.E. (2007). Chapter 18 – Beginning a Homemade Blended Formula. *Homemade Blended Formula Handbook*. Tucson, AZ: Mealtime Notions, LLC.

Klein, M.D. and Morris, S.E. (2007). Chapter 25 – Anatomy of a Recipe. *Homemade blended formula handbook*. Tucson, AZ: Mealtime Notions, LLC.

Klein, M.D. and Morris, S.E. (2007). Appendix B-Calorie Chart. *Homemade Blended Formula Handbook*. Tucson, AZ: Mealtime Notions, LLC.

United States Department of Agriculture. (2005). *Dietary guidelines for Americans*. www.health.gov/dietaryguidelines

United States Department of Agriculture. *National Nutrient Database*. http://www.nal.usda.gov/fnic/foodcomp/search/

United States Department of Agriculture. ChooseMyPlate. http://www.choosemyplate.govnal.usda.gov

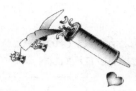

Checklist for Creating a Personal Formula

	Check with your child's physician.
	Determine the list of foods accepted or tolerated by slow introduction (one at a time).
	Estimate the *Calorie Goal* by using the *Daily Calorie Guidelines* or by calculating current commercial formula calories.
	Select appropriate *Homemade Blended Formula Worksheet* based on *Calorie Goal*.
	Choose foods based on the Food Pyramid guidelines equivalents. (Be sure to vary foods daily.)
	Total the calories for each day and add extras, if needed to achieve daily *Calorie Goal*.
	Blend all ingredients adding a little extra fluid if necessary for consistency.
	Measure the total blended volume of the formula.
	Determine the number of calories per ounce/milliliter by dividing the total calories by the total ounces/milliliters.
	Observe and document your child's reaction to the formula.
	Monitor your child's growth

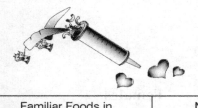

Homemade Blended Formula Tolerance

Familiar Foods in Today's Formula	New Food(s) in Today's Formula	Bowel Movements Consistency	Vomiting Gagging	Discomfort	Other: Rash, Mucus, etc.
		Comments:			

Date _____

Familiar Foods in Today's Formula	New Food(s) in Today's Formula	Bowel Movements Consistency	Vomiting Gagging	Discomfort	Other: Rash, Mucus, etc.
		Comments:			

Date _____

Familiar Foods in Today's Formula	New Food(s) in Today's Formula	Bowel Movements Consistency	Vomiting Gagging	Discomfort	Other: Rash, Mucus, etc.
		Comments:			

Date _____

Familiar Foods in Today's Formula	New Food(s) in Today's Formula	Bowel Movements Consistency	Vomiting Gagging	Discomfort	Other: Rash, Mucus, etc.
		Comments:			

Date _____

Daily Calorie Guidelines

Males   **Females**

Age	Sedentary	Moderately Active	Active	Age	Sedentary	Moderately Active	Active
2 years	1000	1000	1000	2 years	1000	1000	1000
3 years	1000	1400	1400	3 years	1000	1200	1400
4 years	1200	1400	1600	4 years	1200	1400	1400
5 years	1200	1400	1600	5 years	1200	1400	1600
6 years	1400	1600	1800	6 years	1200	1400	1600
7 years	1400	1600	1800	7 years	1200	1600	1800
8 years	1400	1600	2000	8 years	1400	1600	1800
9 years	1600	1800	2000	9 years	1400	1600	1800
10 years	1600	1800	2200	10 years	1400	1800	2000
11 years	1800	2000	2200	11 years	1600	1800	2000
12 years	1800	2200	2400	12 years	1600	2000	2200
13 years	2000	2200	2600	13 years	1600	2000	2200
14 years	2000	2400	2800	14 years	1800	2000	2400
15 years	2200	2600	3000	15 years	1800	2000	2400
16 years	2400	2800	3200	16 years	1800	2000	2400
17 years	2400	2800	3200	17 years	1800	2000	2400
18 years	2400	2800	3200	18 years	1800	2000	2400

Based on My Pyramid Food Intake Pattern Calorie Levels for growth, April 2005   (www.mypyramid.gov)

Homemade Blended Formula Worksheet

Date _____

1000 Calories

Food Group	Tip	Goal: Based on a 1000 Calorie Pattern	List Foods Chosen	Calories
GRAINS	Make at least half your grains whole grains	**3 one-ounce equivalents** (A one-ounce equivalent is about 1 slice of bread, or 1 cup dry cereal, or ½ cup cooked rice, pasta or cereal)		
VEGETABLES	Choose vegetables of different colors for dietary diversity	**1 cup**		
FRUIT	Consider fruits for most choices rather than juices and choose a variety of colors for dietary diversity	**1 cup**		
MILK or MILK SUBSTITUTE	Milks and yogurts tend to blend more easily than cheese	**2 cups**		
MEAT, BEANS, NUTS	Vary choices among meats, poultry, fish, legumes, nuts and seeds	**2 one-ounce equivalents** (A one-ounce equivalent is 1 ounce meat, poultry or fish; 1 egg, 1 tablespoon peanut butter; ½ ounce nuts; or ¼ cup cooked legumes)		
FATS	Choose olive, canola, flax for better health	**3 teaspoons**		
			Subtotal Calories:	
EXTRAS	For children under age 2, add additional fats for brain development. For older children, calories can come from any source.			
			Total Extra Calories:	
			Total Calories:	

Total Calories divided by Total Blended Volume in ounces = Calories Per Ounce OR Total Calories divided by Total Blended Volume in milliliters (mls or ccs) = Calories Per mls or ccs

Adapted from ChooseMyPlate www.choosemyplate.gov. Food recommendations based on United States Department of Agriculture dietary guidelines for Americans (2010) and ChooseMyPlate.

Notes: _____

Homemade Blended Formula Worksheet

Date _____

1200 Calories

Food Group	Tip	Goal: Based on a 1200 Calorie Pattern	List Foods Chosen	Calories
GRAINS	Make at least half your grains whole grains	**4 one-ounce equivalents** (A one-ounce equivalent is about 1 slice of bread, or 1 cup dry cereal, or ½ cup cooked rice, pasta or cereal)		
VEGETABLES	Choose vegetables of different colors for dietary diversity	**1½ cups**		
FRUIT	Consider fruits for most choices rather than juices and choose a variety of colors for dietary diversity	**1 cup**		
MILK or MILK SUBSTITUTE	Milks and yogurts tend to blend more easily than cheese	**2 cups 3 years** **2½ cups 4-8 years**		
MEAT, BEANS, NUTS	Vary choices among meats, poultry, fish, legumes, nuts and seeds	**3 one-ounce equivalents** (A one-ounce equivalent is 1 ounce meat, poultry or fish; 1 egg, 1 tablespoon peanut butter; ½ ounce nuts; or ¼ cup cooked legumes)		
FATS	Choose olive, canola, flax for better health	**4 teaspoons**		
			Subtotal Calories:	
EXTRAS	For children under age 2, add additional fats for brain development. For older children, calories can come from any source.			
			Total Extra Calories:	
			Total Calories:	

Total Calories divided by Total Blended Volume in ounces = Calories Per Ounce OR Total Calories divided by Total Blended Volume in milliliters (mls or ccs) = Calories Per mls or ccs

Adapted from ChooseMyPlate www.choosemyplate.gov. Food recommendations based on United States Department of Agriculture dietary guidelines for Americans (2010) and ChooseMyPlate.

Notes: _____

Homemade Blended Formula Worksheet

Date _____

1400 Calories

Food Group	Tip	Goal: Based on a 1400 Calorie Pattern	List Foods Chosen	Calories
GRAINS	Make at least half your grains whole grains	**5 one-ounce equivalents** (A one-ounce equivalent is about 1 slice of bread, or 1 cup dry cereal, or ½ cup cooked rice, pasta or cereal)		
VEGETABLES	Choose vegetables of different colors for dietary diversity	1½ **cups**		
FRUIT	Consider fruits for most choices rather than juices and choose a variety of colors for dietary diversity	1½ **cups**		
MILK or MILK SUBSTITUTE	Milks and yogurts tend to blend more easily than cheese	2 cups 3 years 2½ cups 4-8 years		
MEAT, BEANS, NUTS	Vary choices among meats, poultry, fish, legumes, nuts and seeds	**4 one-ounce equivalents** (A one-ounce equivalent is 1 ounce meat, poultry or fish; 1 egg, 1 tablespoon peanut butter; ½ ounce nuts; or ¼ cup cooked legumes)		
FATS	Choose olive, canola, flax for better health	**4 teaspoons**		
EXTRAS	For children under age 2, add additional fats for brain development. For older children, calories can come from any source.			
			Subtotal Calories:	
			Total Extra Calories:	
			Total Calories:	

Total Calories divided by Total Blended Volume in ounces = Calories Per Ounce OR Total Calories divided by Total Blended Volume in milliliters (mls or ccs) = Calories Per mls or ccs

Adapted from ChooseMyPlate www.choosemyplate.gov. Food recommendations based on United States Department of Agriculture dietary guidelines for Americans (2010) and ChooseMyPlate.

Notes:_____

Homemade Blended Formula Worksheet

Date _____

Goal:
1600 Calories

Food Group	Tip	Goal: Based on a 1600 Calorie Pattern	List Foods Chosen	Calories
GRAINS	Make at least half your grains whole grains	**5 one-ounce equivalents** (A one-ounce equivalent is about 1 slice of bread, or 1 cup dry cereal, or ½ cup cooked rice, pasta or cereal)		
VEGETABLES	Choose vegetables of different colors for dietary diversity	**2 cups**		
FRUIT	Consider fruits for most choices rather than juices and choose a variety of colors for dietary diversity	**1½ cups**		
MILK or MILK SUBSTITUTE	Milks and yogurts tend to blend more easily than cheese	**2½ cups 4-8 years** **3 cups 9-17+ years**		
MEAT, BEANS, NUTS	Vary choices among meats, poultry, fish, legumes, nuts and seeds	**5 one-ounce equivalents** (A one-ounce equivalent is 1 ounce meat, poultry or fish; 1 egg, 1 tablespoon peanut butter; ½ ounce nuts; or ¼ cup cooked legumes)		
FATS	Choose olive, canola, flax for better health	**5 teaspoons**		
			Subtotal Calories:	
EXTRAS	For older children, calories can come from any source.			
			Total Extra Calories:	
			Total Calories:	

Total Calories divided by Total Blended Volume in ounces = Calories Per Ounce OR Total Calories divided by Total Blended Volume in milliliters (mls or ccs) = Calories Per mls or ccs

Total Calories divided by Total Blended Volume in ounces = Calories Per Ounce OR Total Calories divided by Total Blended Volume in milliliters (mls or ccs) = Calories Per mls or ccs. Food recommendations based on United States Department of Agriculture dietary guidelines for Americans (2010) and ChooseMyPlate..

Notes: _____

Homemade Blended Formula Worksheet

Date _____

1800 Calories

Food Group	Tip	Goal: Based on a 1800 Calorie Pattern	List Foods Chosen	Calories
GRAINS	Make at least half your grains whole grains	**6 one-ounce equivalents** (A one-ounce equivalent is about 1 slice of bread, or 1 cup dry cereal, or ½ cup cooked rice, pasta or cereal)		
VEGETABLES	Choose vegetables of different colors for dietary diversity	**2½ cups**		
FRUIT	Consider fruits for most choices rather than juices and choose a variety of colors for dietary diversity	**1½ cups**		
MILK or MILK SUBSTITUTE	Milks and yogurts tend to blend more easily than cheese	**2½ cups 6-8 years** **3 cups 9-17+ years**		
MEAT, BEANS, NUTS	Vary choices among meats, poultry, fish, legumes, nuts and seeds	**5 one-ounce equivalents** (A one-ounce equivalent is 1 ounce meat, poultry or fish; 1 egg, 1 tablespoon peanut butter; ½ ounce nuts; or ¼ cup cooked legumes)		
FATS	Choose olive, canola, flax for better health	**5 teaspoons**		
			Subtotal Calories:	
EXTRAS	For older children, calories can come from any source.			
			Total Extra Calories:	
			Total Calories:	

Total Calories divided by Total Blended Volume in ounces = Calories Per Ounce OR Total Calories divided by Total Blended Volume in milliliters (mls or ccs) = Calories Per mls or ccs

Adapted from ChooseMyPlate www.choosemyplate.gov. Food recommendations based on United States Department of Agriculture dietary guidelines for Americans (2010) and ChooseMyPlate.

Copyright © 2016 by Mealtime Notions, LLC. Homemade Blended Formula Handbook; Klein and Morris; (520) 829-9635.   This chart may be reproduced for instructional use. This handbook is for educational purposes and should not replace the advice of the physician caring for each child.

Notes: _____

Homemade Blended Formula Worksheet

2000 Calories

Date _____

Food Group	Tip	Goal: Based on a 2000 Calorie Pattern	List Foods Chosen	Calories
GRAINS	Make at least half your grains whole grains	**6 one-ounce equivalents** (A one-ounce equivalent is about 1 slice of bread, or 1 cup dry cereal, or ½ cup cooked rice, pasta or cereal)		
VEGETABLES	Choose vegetables of different colors for dietary diversity	**2½ cups**		
FRUIT	Consider fruits for most choices rather than juices and choose a variety of colors for dietary diversity	**2 cups**		
MILK or MILK SUBSTITUTE	Milks and yogurts tend to blend more easily than cheese	**2½ cups 6-8 years** **3 cups 9-17+ years**		
MEAT, BEANS, NUTS	Vary choices among meats, poultry, fish, legumes, nuts and seeds	**5½ one-ounce equivalents** (A one-ounce equivalent is 1 ounce meat, poultry or fish; 1 egg, 1 tablespoon peanut butter; ½ ounce nuts; or ¼ cup cooked legumes)		
FATS	Choose olive, canola, flax for better health	**6 teaspoons**		
			Subtotal Calories:	
EXTRAS	For older children, calories can come from any source.			
			Total Extra Calories:	
			Total Calories:	

Total Calories divided by Total Blended Volume in ounces = Calories Per Ounce OR Total Calories divided by Total Blended Volume in milliliters (mls or ccs) = Calories Per mls or ccs

Adapted from ChooseMyPlate www.choosemyplate.gov. Food recommendations based on United States Department of Agriculture dietary guidelines for Americans (2010) and ChooseMyPlate.

Notes: _____

Homemade Blended Formula Worksheet

Date _____

2200 Calories

Food Group	Tip	Goal: Based on a 2200 Calorie Pattern	List Foods Chosen	Calories
GRAINS	Make at least half your grains whole grains	**7 one-ounce equivalents** (A one-ounce equivalent is about 1 slice of bread, or 1 cup dry cereal, or ½ cup cooked rice, pasta or cereal)		
VEGETABLES	Choose vegetables of different colors for dietary diversity	**3 cups**		
FRUIT	Consider fruits for most choices rather than juices and choose a variety of colors for dietary diversity	**2 cups**		
MILK or MILK SUBSTITUTE	Milks and yogurts tend to blend more easily than cheese	**3 cups**		
MEAT,BEANS,NUTS	Vary choices among meats, poultry, fish, legumes, nuts and seeds	**6 one-ounce equivalents** (A one-ounce equivalent is 1 ounce meat, poultry or fish; 1 egg; 1 tablespoon peanut butter; ½ ounce nuts; or ¼ cup cooked legumes)		
FATS	Choose olive, canola, flax for better health	**6 teaspoons**		
			Subtotal Calories:	
EXTRAS	For older children, calories can come from any source.			
			Total Extra Calories:	
			Total Calories:	

Total Calories divided by Total Blended Volume in ounces = Calories Per Ounce OR Total Calories divided by Total Blended Volume in milliliters (mls or ccs) = Calories Per mls or ccs

Notes: _____

Homemade Blended Formula Worksheet

Date _____

2400 Calories

Food Group	Tip	Goal: Based on a 2400 Calorie Pattern	List Foods Chosen	Calories
GRAINS	Make at least half your grains whole grains	**8 one-ounce equivalents** (A one-ounce equivalent is about 1 slice of bread, or 1 cup dry cereal, or ½ cup cooked rice, pasta or cereal)		
VEGETABLES	Choose vegetables of different colors for dietary diversity	**3 cups**		
FRUIT	Consider fruits for most choices rather than juices and choose a variety of colors for dietary diversity	**2 cups**		
MILK or MILK SUBSTITUTE	Milks and yogurts tend to blend more easily than cheese	**3 cups**		
MEAT, BEANS, NUTS	Vary choices among meats, poultry, fish, legumes, nuts and seeds	**6½ one-ounce equivalents** (A one-ounce equivalent is 1 ounce meat, poultry or fish; 1 egg, 1 tablespoon peanut butter; ½ ounce nuts; or ¼ cup cooked legumes)		
FATS	Choose olive, canola, flax for better health	**7 teaspoons**		
			Subtotal Calories:	
EXTRAS	For older children, calories can come from any source.		**Total Extra Calories:**	
			Total Calories:	

Total Calories divided by Total Blended Volume in ounces = Calories Per Ounce OR Total Calories divided by Total Blended Volume in milliliters (mls or ccs) = Calories Per mls or ccs

Adapted from ChooseMyPlate www.choosemyplate.gov. Food recommendations based on United States Department of Agriculture dietary guidelines for Americans (2010) and ChooseMyPlate.

Notes: _____

Homemade Blended Formula Worksheet   Date _____

2600 Calories

Food Group	Tip	Goal: Based on a 2600 Calorie Pattern	List Foods Chosen	Calories
GRAINS	Make at least half your grains whole grains	**9 one-ounce equivalents** (A one-ounce equivalent is about 1 slice of bread, or 1 cup dry cereal, or ½ cup cooked rice, pasta or cereal)		
VEGETABLES	Choose vegetables of different colors for dietary diversity	**3½ cups**		
FRUIT	Consider fruits for most choices rather than juices and choose a variety of colors for dietary diversity	**2 cups**		
MILK or MILK SUBSTITUTE	Milks and yogurts tend to blend more easily than cheese	**3 cups**		
MEAT, BEANS, NUTS	Vary choices among meats, poultry, fish, legumes, nuts and seeds	**6½ one-ounce equivalents** (A one-ounce equivalent is 1 ounce meat, poultry or fish; 1 egg, 1 tablespoon peanut butter; ½ ounce nuts; or ¼ cup cooked legumes)		
FATS	Choose olive, canola, flax for better health	**8 teaspoons**		
			Subtotal Calories:	
EXTRAS	For older children, calories can come from any source.			
			Total Extra Calories:	
			Total Calories:	

Total Calories divided by Total Blended Volume in ounces = Calories Per Ounce OR Total Calories divided by Total Blended Volume in milliliters (mls or ccs) = Calories Per mls or ccs

Adapted from ChooseMyPlate www.choosemyplate.gov. Food recommendations based on United States Department of Agriculture dietary guidelines for Americans (2010) and ChooseMyPlate.

Notes: _____

Homemade Blended Formula Worksheet

Date _____

2800 Calories

Food Group	Tip	Goal: Based on a 2800 Calorie Pattern	List Foods Chosen	Calories
GRAINS	Make at least half your grains whole grains	**10 one-ounce equivalents** (A one-ounce equivalent is about 1 slice of bread, or 1 cup dry cereal, or ½ cup cooked rice, pasta or cereal)		
VEGETABLES	Choose vegetables of different colors for dietary diversity	**3½ cups**		
FRUIT	Consider fruits for most choices rather than juices and choose a variety of colors for dietary diversity	**2½ cups**		
MILK or MILK SUBSTITUTE	Milks and yogurts tend to blend more easily than cheese	**3 cups**		
MEAT, BEANS, NUTS	Vary choices among meats, poultry, fish, legumes, nuts and seeds	**7 one-ounce equivalents** (A one-ounce equivalent is 1 ounce meat, poultry or fish; 1 egg, 1 tablespoon peanut butter; ½ ounce nuts; or ¼ cup cooked legumes)		
FATS	Choose olive, canola, flax for better health	**8 teaspoons**		
EXTRAS	For older children, calories can come from any source.			
			Subtotal Calories:	
			Total Extra Calories:	
			Total Calories:	

Total Calories divided by Total Blended Volume in ounces = Calories Per Ounce OR Total Calories divided by Total Blended Volume in milliliters (mls or ccs) = Calories Per mls or ccs

Copyright © 2016 by Mealtime Notions, LLC. Homemade Blended Formula Handbook; Klein and Morris; (520) 829-9635. This chart may be reproduced for instructional use. This handbook is for educational purposes and should not replace the advice of the physician caring for each child.
Adapted from ChooseMyPlate www.choosemyplate.gov. Food recommendations based on United States Department of Agriculture dietary guidelines for Americans (2010) and ChooseMyPlate.

Notes:_____

Homemade Blended Formula Worksheet

Date _____

3000 Calories

Food Group	Tip	Goal: Based on a 3000 Calorie Pattern	List Foods Chosen	Calories
GRAINS	Make at least half your grains whole grains	**10 one-ounce equivalents** (A one-ounce equivalent is about 1 slice of bread, or 1 cup dry cereal, or ½ cup cooked rice, pasta or cereal)		
VEGETABLES	Choose vegetables of different colors for dietary diversity	**4 cups**		
FRUIT	Consider fruits for most choices rather than juices and choose a variety of colors for dietary diversity	**2½ cups**		
MILK or MILK SUBSTITUTE	Milks and yogurts tend to blend more easily than cheese	**3 cups**		
MEAT, BEANS, NUTS	Vary choices among meats, poultry, fish, legumes, nuts and seeds	**7 one-ounce equivalents** (A one-ounce equivalent is 1 ounce meat, poultry or fish; 1 egg, 1 tablespoon peanut butter; ½ ounce nuts; or ¼ cup cooked legumes)		
FATS	Choose olive, canola, flax for better health	**10 teaspoons**		
			Subtotal Calories:	
EXTRAS	For older children, calories can come from any source.			
			Total Extra Calories:	
			Total Calories:	

Total Calories divided by Total Blended Volume in ounces = Calories Per Ounce OR Total Calories divided by Total Blended Volume in milliliters (mls or ccs) = Calories Per mls or ccs

Notes: _____

Homemade Blended Formula Worksheet

3200 Calories

Date _____

Food Group	Tip	Goal: Based on a 3200 Calorie Pattern	List Foods Chosen	Calories
GRAINS	Make at least half your grains whole grains	**10 one-ounce equivalents** (A one-ounce equivalent is about 1 slice of bread, or 1 cup dry cereal, or ½ cup cooked rice, pasta or cereal)		
VEGETABLES	Choose vegetables of different colors for dietary diversity	**4 cups**		
FRUIT	Consider fruits for most choices rather than juices and choose a variety of colors for dietary diversity	**2½ cups**		
MILK or MILK SUBSTITUTE	Milks and yogurts tend to blend more easily than cheese	**3 cups**		
MEAT, BEANS, NUTS	Vary choices among meats, poultry, fish, legumes, nuts and seeds	**7 one-ounce equivalents** (A one-ounce equivalent is 1 ounce meat, poultry or fish; 1 egg; 1 tablespoon peanut butter; ½ ounce nuts; or ¼ cup cooked legumes)		
FATS	Choose olive, canola, flax for better health	**11 teaspoons**		
			Subtotal Calories:	
EXTRAS	For older children, calories can come from any source.			
			Total Extra Calories:	
			Total Calories:	

Total Calories divided by Total Blended Volume in ounces = Calories Per Ounce OR Total Calories divided by Total Blended Volume in milliliters (mls or ccs) = Calories Per mls or ccs

Notes: _____

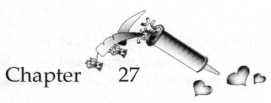

Chapter 27

Preparation Tips from Parents

Suzanne Evans Morris, Ph.D, CCC

Preparation of a homemade blended formula often involves a great deal of trial and error. It's much easier to decide which foods are needed to create a nutritious diet for a child than it is to fine-tune the diet so that it passes easily through a feeding tube and provides a volume of food the child can handle comfortably.

Dozens of parents have contributed their personal experiences to the *Homemade Blended Formula Handbook*. Some have contributed chapters. Many others have contributed their questions, thoughts and experiences exploring and creating homemade blended formulas for their children. They offered specific and practical preparation tips through personal discussion and in response to a series of questionnaires. This chapter summarizes their personal learning.

Nutritional Content Tips

- It's important to know how many calories and how much of each nutrient your child needs, according to her weight and age. Ask your dietitian for this specific information, in addition to specific formula recommendations.

- A book that provides the exact number of calories and the amount of protein, fat and carbohydrate for each food is helpful. This allows you to monitor the overall nutritional content of the formulas you're creating or modifying.

- Once you and your dietitian have developed an appropriate diet and core menus, you can modify the homemade blended formulas just as you would modify the daily diet of an orally fed child. For most children you don't have to count every calorie and nutrient that goes into the formula, as long as you use common sense and an overall perspective of what your child needs in order to grow and be healthy.

- You can create a spreadsheet in your computer or use an online nutritional program with your dietitian to calculate calories and nutrients as you create variations on the core formulas.

- Don't worry if each batch of formula varies a bit in content and nutrition because this is the natural way of eating. It's important to remember that children's diets vary a great deal from meal to meal and day to day. Over a period of several days they get what their bodies need. This is a model that has been very helpful in thinking about variations in homemade blended formulas.

- There are a number of books specifically written for parents who want to make homemade baby foods for their infants and toddlers. Many offer invaluable information on nutrition, preparation and ingredients for the baby food. These suggestions can be modified by adding a nutritious liquid so the blend will be thin enough to pass through the feeding tube.

- To get an idea of the amounts children and adults eat, blend up a submarine sandwich! Add enough liquid to make it a smooth mixture that could pass through a syringe and tube. This makes enough food to fill three to four 60 ml syringes!

- Buy good nutritious food. If you have access and can afford it, buy organic vegetables and fruits, as well as meats and eggs. Locally grown organic foods often have more nutrients because they've been ripened on the vine or tree, rather than picked green and shipped across the country.

- Consider purchasing organic baby foods if you're using ready-prepared pureed foods. These are available year-round and are free of pesticides and other chemicals.

- Children don't need meat. They do need adequate protein, which can be provided in any number of ways, including powdered protein from a variety of commercially available sources (bean protein, pea protein, egg protein, whey, rice, soy), and other high-protein foods such as tofu, legumes, grains, eggs and many vegetables.

- The dark meat of the chicken contains more fat and adds more calories than white meat. Purchasing boneless and skinless chicken thighs makes it easier and faster to prepare.

- Vary the foods you add to the diet according to the child's daily health needs. When a child is constipated, add more blended fruit or prune juice. When a child is on antibiotics, consider adding more yogurt containing probiotic cultures.

- Try each new food separately and in very small amounts. You can blend the new food with a small amount of milk or formula and give it in increasing amounts for a few days to see if there are any negative reactions. Look for rashes, hives, diarrhea, constipation, emotional or gastrointestinal changes. This way, you won't make a large batch of something your child can't tolerate and have to throw it out.

Food Preparation Tips

Mealtime Patterns and Strategies

- Consider making a single day's worth of a "recipe" at a time. The recipe contains meats, vegetables, cereals, dairy, oils, fruits and miscellaneous vitamins or supplements. Change the recipe pattern or rotate different fruits, vegetables, etc., to provide variety, following the overall recommendations of nutrients and servings in ChooseMyPlate.

- Consider making two different meal recipes for the day. The breakfast meal has a base of cereal, fruit and yogurt. The lunch and dinner meals have a base of vegetables and meat or other protein. The specific foods in these recipes vary during the day and more closely mimic the types of meals served to oral eaters.

- You can offer your child a plate at the beginning of the meal that contains a variation of the same foods the rest of the family is eating. This gives an opportunity for the child to orally taste and sample as much of the food as possible. Blend the foods from the family meal and give them to the child by tube.

- Many children are able to taste their tube-food as it goes into the stomach. They recognize particular tastes and foods when they're offered orally later. When possible, create a meal mixture that tastes good. It should be blander for infants and toddlers, and more varied and spicier for older children

Preparation Strategies

- Buy fresh vegetables, cook or steam them in the pot with a small amount of water. Remember to include both green and yellow vegetables because each contains different vitamins. You can cook all the vegetables together or cook each one separately. When they're soft, put in the blender and make very smooth puree, with no bumps or lumps in it.

- If liquid is needed, add the water that the vegetables cooked in. This water contains many of the nutrients that originally were in the vegetables. The resulting mixture should be thin enough to go through the tube or pour into ice cube trays for storage.

- You initially can make a thick mixture and then thin it with milk, juice or broth to a consistency that will go through the syringe and tube. After thinning, the ideal consistency should be not quite as thick as pudding, but thinner than cake batter.

- Fill the blender half full and blend the mixture while the food is warm. Add a small amount of liquid at a time. You always can add more, but you can't subtract it. If you desire a thick, well-blended puree, stop intermittently to stir the food with a spatula. This makes it easier to get just the right amount of liquid to obtain a consistently smooth puree.

- Thoroughly wash all fresh fruits and vegetables before you cook them or add them to the blended formula. You can purchase a commercial fruit-and-vegetable wash that's formulated to remove wax, oily pesticides, soil and chemicals from the surface of the fruit or vegetable.

- If using organically grown fruits such as apples or peaches, you don't have to peel them if you're using a high-powered blender (such as the Vita-Mix or Blenctec brand) that will liquefy the peels. Many of the nutrients lie between the skin and the fruit, and are lost when peeled. Peel non-organic fruits to eliminate pesticides and other chemicals in the skin of the fruit.

- Boil chicken or turkey in a pot of water until it's very soft, and then grind the chicken and broth in the blender until it looks like a latte smoothie. This process takes a while but the meat will last for a month or more, depending on how many cubes of meat you'll use daily.

- If you don't have a high-powered blender or don't want to cook and puree meats, buy commercial pureed baby food meats. This is much easier than trying to prepare meat in a regular blender.

- Canned or jarred or frozen pumpkin, squash, mango, papaya, tomato puree and applesauce can be used to cut down on pureeing time and add variety during the winter and spring months, when the selection of fresh fruits and vegetables is more limited.

- Although you can use baby cereal for the grains group, it's much less expensive and more nutritious to make a porridge or congee from whole ground grains (i.e. brown rice, rolled oats, barley, millet). Use a crock pot or slow cooker to cook the whole grains in water,

then use the blender to blend the porridge into the puree. Add water if needed to create a smooth mixture. It's very easy to prepare the grain mixture and then freeze a large batch into ice cubes, which you can use as needed.

- Cook foods such as frozen vegetables and powdered grains in either vegetable broth or fruit juice to increase the calories and nutrients.

Food Properties

- Brown rice blends more easily and becomes less like a paste than white rice.

- Avocado is an excellent source of fat and should be used uncooked.

- Avocados and bananas should be fresh and added the day of the meal.

- It's very efficient to use only de-boned chicken. If you use a whole chicken, it's easy to accidentally get cartilage and bone in the meat mixture. Then you either have to strain the whole batch or live with occasional tube blockages.

- Milk often "grows" when you blend it. You get lots of problems with bubbles, which can cause a child to develop more gas. It also increases the volume of the food and takes up more space in the stomach. If your recipe includes milk, soymilk, yogurt or formula, add it just before serving and blend it very slowly for a short period of time, to mix it with the rest of the food.

- Don't add milk or commercial formulas to a mixture that you're going to freeze. Most formula manufacturers specifically warn against freezing their products.

- If you pour frothy formula into a container that can be sealed with a vacuum sealer, and then extract the air, the froth will nearly disappear.

- Certain foods thicken the mixture. Be careful not to combine many of these foods in the same recipe. Some foods that thicken a mixture include, pasta and other wheat products, oatmeal, bananas, potatoes, blueberries and avocado.

- Fresh blueberries and cranberries blend in a recipe more easily than dried blueberries or cranberries.

- Potatoes don't freeze well. If you include them in a recipe that will be frozen, put them in the blender to smooth them out before serving.

- Acidic foods such as oranges, grapefruit, lemons, limes and tomatoes can interact with milk and cause it to curdle when the foods aren't cooked. This doesn't happen when the mixture is cooked.

- If grinding your own whole uncooked grains, grind them in an electric coffee bean grinder, then cook for a minute or two on the stove, like a porridge, using one part milled grain to five parts liquid.

- Nuts, seeds and chewable vitamins blend more easily if you grind them in the coffee bean grinder before adding them to the blender.

- Fresh flaxseed can be a challenge to blend because the seeds will stick in the feeding button or tube if they're not fully crushed and ground. Add water or Pedialyte® to the blender and then add the flaxseed. Blend the two ingredients on "low" for several minutes. Turn off the blender and let the seeds fall to the bottom of the blender and then blend everything again.

- Some foods are harder to blend into a smooth mixture than others. Spinach may be stringy. Fresh corn may leave small pieces of the skin. Small seeds of raspberries and other berries may not be completely pureed. A great deal depends upon the power and efficiency of the blender you're using.

- Slow-cooked congee moves through the tube best if it's blended after it is cooked.

Food Storage

- You may prefer to cook and prepare the foods for homemade blended formulas ahead of time. It may require an hour or two once a week to prepare the food. If you freeze the blended mixture, it's available to provide the variety for different recipes each day.

- There are at least three ways to store pureed food for future use:

    Blend enough of the child's total recipe to last one or two days and keep it in jars in the refrigerator. A formula can be refrigerated for up to 48 hours.

    Blend larger amounts of the child's total recipe and freeze a full day's menu in each glass jar.

    Blend each food separately and freeze in ice cube trays. Store each food in a separate re-sealable freezer bag or disposable plastic container.

- Each ice cube will hold a serving size of 1.5 to 2 tablespoons of food.

- After preparing the food and placing it in the ice cube trays, cover the tray with foil and put it in the freezer for 24 hours. Twist the ice cube trays so that the cubes pop out and store them in re-sealable plastic bags. If the ice cubes don't pop out easily, leave the tray out on the counter for 10-15 minutes.

- Label each freezer bag with the date the food was prepared and frozen.

- It's very efficient to combine frozen food cubes into daily meal packs. From the larger bag of separate frozen food cubes, assemble daily meal bags that contain the exact amount and assortment of foods needed for one day. For example, each daily bag might contain 1 meat cube, 1 split pea cube, 2 green vegetable cubes,

2 yellow/red vegetable cubes and 3 porridge cubes. Keep the daily packs in the freezer. When you're putting a meal together in the morning, take out one daily pack, put the cubes in a glass dish and thaw them in the microwave. It usually takes about 15 minutes to unfreeze the bag.

- Place thawed food cubes in the blender; add the non-frozen components of the formula. Blend at a low speed to mix all ingredients and obtain the appropriate amount of thickness.

- In order to preserve the nutrients in fresh fruits and vegetables, add uncooked or lightly steamed to the slow-cooked frozen foods on the day of the meal.

- Oil may separate in the formula mixture when it's stored in the refrigerator for several days or frozen. This depends upon the amount of oil and the food base to which it's added. To solve this problem, blend the oil into the formula on the day of the meal rather than ahead of time.

- Cook a mixture of meat and grain in bulk for about an hour, and freeze in 2-cup portions. Take out one portion and let it thaw before putting it in the blender. In this way you can make up a package of meat (such as chicken livers, pork tenders, turkey breasts) and mix with the appropriate amount of grain and cook them together, which often is easier than cooking and freezing meats and grains separately.

- Freezing food in jars or cubes makes it easier to rotate different foods into the child's diet and reduce the tendency to use the same foods every day.

- Like other baby foods, don't leave the formula at room temperature. Put it in the refrigerator or in an insulated lunch bag with an ice pack when traveling. Warm the food before giving it to your child.

- Warm the formula after it's blended to pop any air bubbles in the mixture. Refrigerate it until needed.

Equipment

Syringes & Tubes

- Use olive oil or spray the syringe plunger tip with a spray oil (such as PAM®) to lubricate the end of the plunger and make it easier to slide through the syringe as food is pushed through the tube.

- Assemble the syringe by inserting the plunger into the syringe. Push the plunger all the way to the end until there's no air left in the syringe. Put the end of the syringe into the prepared food and slowly pull the plunger up. Make sure there's no air in the syringe. When the syringe is full, turn the syringe up and *very slowly* push the air out. Watch out for the food shooting up in the air! You'll get better with time, but the flying food often is part of the learning experience. Connect the syringe to the extension tube and push the food through the tube until both syringe and the tube are filled with the food. Push the food in very slowly and watch for any signs of discomfort. Adjust your speed and volume to meet your child's needs.

- Practice pushing food through the tube into a bowl or jar until you have a physical perception of how much pressure to use. Work toward moving the food slowly and gently through the tube. You'll get slightly more resistance and need to use a little bit more pressure when you're pushing the food through a feeding button.

- Flush the feeding button with water within an hour after feeding. It's ideal to do this immediately after the meal if the child's stomach can handle the additional liquid.

- Homemade blended formulas stick to tubes and syringes more than commercial formulas. It's essential to take time to clean them well.

Use hot soapy water and a baby-bottle brush. You also can dip them in a dilute bleach and water solution for further sterilizing. Wash syringes and tubes immediately after using them so food doesn't dry in them.

- Using the dull side of a knife, run it along the connector tube while running hot water through it. This method will clean even the dirtiest tube. To clean the tip of the connector tube, use pipe cleaners from a craft store.

- Keep a supply of syringes, tubes and an extra feeding button on hand. Some parents find that these wear out slightly faster with a homemade formula than they do with a commercial formula. Others have seen no difference at all.

Blenders & Strainers

- The type of blender you use will depend upon the type of food you wish to prepare and include in your child's recipe. A regular kitchen blender can be used very successfully when pureeing softer fruits, vegetables and grains. It also can be used to mix up the daily formula from frozen food cubes and other ready-made food components. It's all you need if your formula consists primarily of commercial baby foods and formula. A high powered specialized blender such as the Vita-Mix is ideal if you are preparing more complex meals, especially if you wish to include vegetables such as corn, fruits with peelings and freshly prepared meat.

- If using a regular kitchen blender, filter pureed food through a fine sieve or grease spatter shield to remove pieces that might clog the feeding button and tube. Discard bits of fiber that you can't push through the strainer with a heavy rubber spatula.

- With a regular kitchen blender, you can blend some meat successfully by blending the mixture twice.

- It's much easier to prevent pieces of bone, cartilage and fiber from getting stuck in the tube than to fix it later. However, if something does get stuck, you can remove it by the following procedure: Unhook the tube from your child and insert the syringe tip in the end of the tube that usually goes into the feeding button. Push the food back out the tube to remove any chunks that made it through the blender. It's messy, but not impossible.

- Vita-Mix Corporation offers a Medical Needs Discount Program, which is available to all eligible candidates. This program offers patients an opportunity to purchase a factory reconditioned machine at a significant discount. If you feel that you qualify for this discount, please contact Vita-Mix Corporation for details. Eligibility will be determined by Vita-Mix Corporation. Call 1-800-848-2649 or e-mail household@vitamix.com for assistance ; reference this code: ***07-0036-0011***.

Pumps

- Parents have reported a wide variety of experiences using a homemade blended formula with a feeding pump. Some pumps and mixture consistencies work well. Others do not. Kangaroo® and Zevex® pumps have worked successfully for many.

- To pass through a pump, the blended food can be a bit thicker than formula, but shouldn't be too much thicker. It may take some time to find exactly the right thickness that works for a given pump. If the consistency isn't right, the pump will sound a warning alarm.

- If the formula is too thick, the "no flow in" alarm sounds. This can be remedied by thinning the formula with a liquid.

- If there are air bubbles in the formula or if the formula is too cold, the "no-food" alarm sounds. You can solve the problem by adding a few drops of an anti-gas preparation (i.e. Mylanta® or Simethicone®) to the formula. Warming the formula also will get rid of the air bubbles because heat will pop them.

- The thicker formula may cause the pump to deliver less total food at one time. For example if a 500 ml bag is filled to the top and the total amount (dose) is set for 490 ml per hour, there's still some formula left at the end of this time. If the same amount of a thinner formula is given at the same rate, it flows at the 490 ml rate specified on the dial.

- A homemade blended formula should be given by feeding pump only if the "meal" is presented in less than two hours. It should not be given overnight since the food could spoil. Keeping the formula cool with ice (as some parents do with commercial formulas) can cause it to thicken and not pass through the pump and tube.

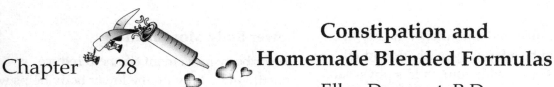

Chapter 28

Constipation and Homemade Blended Formulas

Ellen Duperret, R.D.

Constipation is a very common complaint in children with developmental, gastrointestinal, immune system, and/or neurological conditions. Homemade blended formulas can contribute substantially to improved bowel function and reduce the impact of constipation.

Constipation can be defined as infrequent bowel movements or hard, small stools; difficult or painful evacuation of stools; and encopresis (voluntary or involuntary soiling of the underwear).

Constipation is most generally understood as a delay or difficulty with bowel movements. The term "delay" varies with age. During the first week of life, infants pass an average of four stools per day. (Formula-fed infants have more bowel movements than breast-fed infants.) By age two, children have about two daily and by age four, they average one per day.

A "normal" stooling pattern varies from child to child. One child might have a pattern of several stools daily, whereas another might have a pattern of one every other day, or every third day. If a child usually goes every third day and passes the stool without difficulty or pain, then it's not an issue. However, if there's a hard stool every third day that's painful to pass, then this is a concern. This pattern can result in a fear of elimination, and a decreased appetite.

Children fed by tube can have difficulties with constipation. Any child with chronic constipation should see a physician so that any medical issues can be addressed. Certain medications may have gastrointestinal side effects that cause constipation. Let's explore some of the factors that contribute to constipation, and some ideas for relieving it.

Dietary Support

Many parents report that their children are less constipated after incorporating more homemade blended foods through the tube. Many people adequately control constipation through dietary changes and by providing foods high in fiber. Fiber, the indigestible part of plants, produces a bulky stool, which passes through the colon more easily. It works like a sponge, pulling water through the intestinal wall into the colon. A lack of sufficient fiber in the diet will cause the stools to be harder and more difficult to eliminate. Many tube fed children lack fiber in their diets; the change to a homemade blended formula offers the opportunity to add fiber-rich foods.

There are a number of foods that are offered in an oral diet to help with constipation. These same foods can be added to the homemade blended formula. It's important to remember to introduce only one new food at a time, and start with a small amount.

A common beginning food would be dried plums (commonly called prunes). They can be offered as a juice by tube, or as a part of a blended formula diet or recipe. The following foods might be added gradually to the tube feeding to increase the fiber content of the blend: cooked whole grains, soft cooked beans, bran, flaxseeds, vegetables and fruits.

Fiber Recommendations

How much fiber should a child consume? Current recommendations for children are as follows:

Recommended Dietary Allowance for Fiber for Children*	
Age	Dietary Fiber
1-3 years	19 grams per day
4-8 years	25 grams per day
9-13 years, males	31 grams per day
14-18 years, males	38 grams per day
9-13 years, females	26 grams per day
14-18 years females	26 grams per day

*Based on 2002, the Food and Nutrition Board of the National Academy of Sciences Research Council issued Dietary Reference Intakes (DRI) for fiber.

137

These are recommended amounts of dietary fiber and they should be adapted to each individual child's needs. Check with your child's physician about adding other remedies for significant constipation issues.

Fluids

Fiber without adequate fluids can worsen constipation. Sufficient fluids and free water are needed in the diet for the fiber to be effective. Providing adequate fluid intake is one of the major advantages of tube feeding. Children who are unable to drink liquids by mouth because of oral motor or swallowing difficulties would become dehydrated if they didn't have the physical support of a feeding tube.

Milk, water, broth and vegetable juices are typically used in the preparation of homemade blended formulas. These provide some additional fluids, however they may not be sufficient to meet fluid requirements. For this reason, parents and dietitians must plan to offer separate tube feedings of water ("free water") to meet the child's hydration needs. Generally, it's not recommended to add water to the diet of an infant under 9-12 months of age. (Ask your physician.) However, as the child consumes more solid foods after 9-12 months, small amounts of water and juice are added to the diet to increase fluids.

Check the guidelines for fluid needs for infants and children to make sure that the child is getting an adequate amount. Some children are on concentrated commercial formulas, which contain less water than normally diluted formulas.

Children who do not have feeding difficulties are typically offered drinks of water between meals. Similarly, many families give a water bolus 30 minutes before a tube meal. It's important to remember to give water through the tube (or by mouth if possible) at other times during the day. Avoid giving soda or other sugary beverages for fluids, as they're empty calories with low nutritional value. Excessive cow's milk intake can cause constipation and, for some, replacing milk with other fluids and food alleviates hard stools.

Lower Body Movement

Lower body movement can help reduce constipation. Moving the lower body helps with peristalsis of the intestines, thus allowing the food or fecal matter to pass through more easily. Lack of lower body movement may be due to a lack of exercise or a developmental disability involving gross motor delays. Low muscle tone, or hypotonia (as in Down Syndrome) and increased muscle tone, or hypertonia (as in some types of cerebral palsy), are associated with increased incidence of constipation. When children have hypotonia, the low tone can also exist in the gastrointestinal tract and muscles of the abdominal wall. The low tone can make it more difficult for the child to have the sustained muscle endurance needed for proper elimination. On the other hand, hypertonia can delay the passage of stool by creating too much tension in muscles around the lower body, making efficient, sustained elimination challenging.

Parents can offer massages and leg exercises to children with tone issues, or they can make sure there's some time each day for more active children to go on walks or run around the backyard, park or playground. Children who spend most of their time sitting are much more likely to be constipated than their active counterparts.

Medications

Sometimes increased fiber, fluids and lower body movement aren't enough to alleviate constipation. In that case, a physician may need to prescribe a medication to help the child have regular bowel movements that won't be difficult or painful to pass. Medications used to treat constipation include: bulking agents, stool softeners, osmotic agents, irritant laxatives, and enemas/suppositories. Mineral oil is not recommended for long-term use because it decreases the absorption of fat-soluble vitamins (A, D, E, and K). Talk to your physician about the proper medication regime for constipation if the above approaches aren't solving the problem.

Recipe Support

The following recipes have been created to help with constipation.

Tasty Fiber Recipe

⅓ cup raisins
6 pitted dried plums (prunes)
½ orange, peeled
½ apple, unpeeled
2 Tbsp prune juice
2 Tbsp orange juice

Puree in blender for 2 minutes and store in refrigerator. This paste can be added to a blended formula mixture for tube fed children. It typically is spread on toast or used as a topping with yogurt or ice cream for oral eaters. Adults use 1-2 tablespoons per day, as needed for bowel support. Children typically are started with 1 teaspoon a day. The amount may be increased to 1 tablespoon a day as tolerated, depending on the child's reaction and the effect on the constipation.

Fiber Jello

½ cup applesauce
1 cup water
½ cup apple juice
2 Tbsp psyllium powder (or Metamucil®)
1 box of powdered flavored gelatin (any flavor, regular or sugar-free)

Mix all ingredients and pour into an 8-inch square pan. Chill until set. More, or less water may be needed to get a gelatin that sets. When firm, cut into 1-inch cubes. Start serving one or two cubes per day and increase until a soft stool is passed. More psyllium may be added to the recipe if needed.

For additional information on management of constipation in children see:

Klein, M.D. and Morris, S.E. (2007). Chapter 16 – Homemade Blended Formulas and Hydration. *Homemade Blended Formula Handbook.* Tucson, AZ: Mealtime Notions, LLC.

Klein, M.D. and Morris, S.E. (2007). Appendix E–Food Sources of Dietary Fiber. *Homemade Blended Formula Handbook.* Tucson, AZ: Mealtime Notions, LLC.

Wilson, V., Wick, N. (2007) Constipation in Children. *EMedicineHealth.* http://www.emedicinehealth.com/script/main/art.asp?articlekey=59429&pf=3&page=2

For additional information on massage for children with constipation see:

Drehobl, K.F., Fuhr, M.G. and Erhardt, R. (2000). *Pediatric Massage for the Child with Special Needs, Revised Edition.* Austin, TX: Pro-Ed.

Morris, S.E. and Klein, M.D. (2000) Chapter 22–The Child Who has Gastrointestinal Discomfort. *Pre-Feeding Skills – A Comprehensive Resource for Mealtime Development 2nd Ed.* Austin, TX: Pro-Ed.

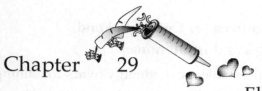

Chapter 29

Special Diets and Homemade Blended Formula

Ellen Duperret, R.D. and Jude Trautlein, R.D.

Many children who receive tube feedings for some or all of their nutrition require therapeutic diets. With physician approval, homemade blended formulas can be based on the same guidelines as those for orally fed children.

What is a Special Diet?

A special diet is one that involves the addition, substitution, elimination or restriction of certain foods for optimal health. Special diets are followed because of food sensitivity, or for management of a disease or metabolic disorder. Some families choose special diets because of nutritional preferences, not for medical necessity.

Children with chronic constipation may have extra fluids and fiber added to the diet. Liver disorders may require the substitution of more easily digested fats. Gluten is eliminated from the diet of children who have celiac disease. Renal disease may require restriction of protein, fluids or minerals. Many families whose children have diagnoses on the autism spectrum may choose to eliminate gluten and dairy products from their child's diet.

The ketogenic diet for seizure control is a precise high-fat, low-carbohydrate diet that must be ordered by a physician and individually designed and monitored by a registered dietitian (R.D.). The child's food must be carefully weighed and restricted to what has been determined by the R.D. The food can be offered orally, or blended and given by tube.

Diets for metabolic disorders generally require the use of medical foods (specialized commercial formulas), and close supervision by a registered dietitian specializing in metabolic disorders. The R.D. can help a family decide if a homemade blended formula is possible for their child.

Food Sensitivity

Food sensitivities are the main reason for children to be on special diets.

Sensitivity includes food allergies and intolerances. Allergies are an adverse immune reaction to a food, generally a protein, which is harmless to most other people. Intake of the offending food may cause a rash, hives, eczema, nasal congestion, fatigue, reflux, vomiting, emotional irritability, breathing difficulties or even anaphylactic shock. The most common food allergies are cow's milk, wheat, corn, soy, peanuts, tree nuts, fish and seafood. Food intolerance may be caused by a digestion problem or an enzyme deficiency.

Because tube fed children often have sensitive digestive systems, it's important to introduce new foods carefully to rule out allergies and intolerances. This is why we advocate presenting one new food at a time when beginning a homemade blended diet, just as is done when offering new foods to oral eaters transitioning from breast milk or formula to solid foods.

Introducing only one new food every three to five days and then watching for symptoms makes it possible to determine which foods are tolerated or need to be avoided.

Milk Allergy

Milk is the most common food sensitivity in children. They can be allergic to the protein in milk (milk allergy), or they can have an intolerance to the sugar in milk (lactose intolerance). Those with a milk allergy must avoid the milk proteins, casein and whey. Milk allergy symptoms vary from child to child and may include abdominal pain, reflux, vomiting, diarrhea, eczema, hives and even blood in the stool. To eliminate food with milk protein, read the label carefully for foods and food components, which contain casein and whey.

141

Milk (Lactose) Intolerance

Lactose intolerance is the body's inability to digest lactose, the sugar in milk. Symptoms include abdominal pain, bloating, gas and loose, watery stools. Most people who suffer from lactose intolerance can comfortably consume foods containing small amounts of lactose such as yogurt or cheese. There are lactose-reduced and lactose-free milks available, as well as products that aid the digestion of lactose.

Gluten Intolerance

Gluten intolerance is a result of an immune response to the gluten protein. This intolerance causes damage to the small bowel, which interferes with nutrient absorption. Symptoms include abdominal bloating, vomiting and growth failure. Management requires the elimination of all foods containing gluten from the diet, including wheat, oats, rye and barley.

Food Sources for Common Food Allergies and Intolerances

It's often a challenge to identify foods containing milk protein, gluten, corn and soy protein by reading labels. These food components are present in a great many foods by many different names. For example one would expect sweeteners such as corn syrup and corn sugar to contain corn. However, dextrose, fructose and maltodextrin are also sweeteners based on corn.

Homemade Blended Formulas

Children following special diets, whether for treatment or by family choice, can choose to follow a homemade blended diet with the support of their physicians and dietitians. The diet prescription will help the family determine where their child's homemade blended diet can fit along the continuum of food choices.

For additional information on food allergies and their management see:

Allergy Resources International. *Allergy advisor: Allergy and Intolerance Software* http://allergyadvisor.com/

Joneja, J. (2003) *Dealing with Food Allergies: A Practical Guide to Detecting Culprit Foods and Eating a Healthy, Enjoyable Diet.* Boulder, CO: Bull Publishing Company.

Klein, M.D. and Morris, S.E. (2007). Appendix Q–Food Sources for Common Food Allergies and Intolerances. *Homemade Blended Formula Handbook.* Tucson:, AZ. Mealtime Notions, LLC.

Melina, V. Stephaniak, J. and Aronson, D. (2004). *Food Allergy Survival Guide: Delicious Recipes & Complete Nutrition.* Summertown, TN: Healthy Living Publications.

Rapp, D. (1991) *Is This Your Child: Discovering and Treating Unrecognized Allergies.* New York, NY: Harper Paperbacks.

For additional information on the gluten- and casein-free diet see:

Case, S. (2006). *Gluten-Free Diet: A Comprehensive Resource Guide.* Regina, SK : Case Nutrition Consulting

Lewis, L. (1998) *Special Diets for Special Kids.* Arlington, TX: Future Horizons

Celiac Sprue Association. *Gluten-Free Diet: Grains and Flours Glossary* www.csaceliacs.org/glutengrains.php

Celiac.com. *Celiac Disease and Gluten-Free Diet Information.* www.celiac.com

GFCF Diet Support Group. The GFCF Diet: Gluten Free Casein Free. www.gfcfdiet.com

Gluten Free Mall: Gluten-Free Foods for Celiac Disease Diets. www.glutenfreemall.com

For additional information on the ketogenic diet see:

Freeman, J.M., Freeman, J., Kelly, M. (2000) *The Ketogenic Diet: A Treatment for Epilepsy, 3rd Ed.* New York, NY: Demos Publishing, Inc.

Amorde-Spalding, K. et al., (1997). The Use of the Ketogenic Diet for Seizure Control in Children. *Nutrition Focus Newsletter.* May-June. http://depts.washington.edu/chdd/ucedd/ctu5/nutritionnews_5.html

Epilepsy Foundation. *General Information About the Ketogenic Diet.* http://www.epilepsyfoundation.org/answerplace/Medical/treatment/diet/

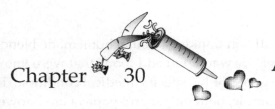

Chapter 30

Mother's Perspective:
A Child's Special Dietary Needs

Tina Valente

My son Joey, nine, has a genetic liver disease. He also has a number of gastrointestinal issues that complicate his life, including severe reflux, slow stomach emptying and malabsorption of fats and vitamins. Eating has been difficult for Joey since birth and he received a gastrostomy tube at nine months of age.

An aspect of Joey's life that's often difficult for our family is the special dietary and feeding needs that result from his serious medical condition. Although it's been a bit of a challenge, a homemade blended formula is one of the ways we've found to support our child's growth, health and well being.

Joey's History

Every family I meet has their own unique story and ours is no exception. Joey was diagnosed in early infancy with a liver disease called Alagille's syndrome (AGS). It's a very rare disorder characterized by a reduced number of small bile ducts within the liver, as well as abnormalities in other organs including the heart, eyes, spine, kidneys, lungs and pancreas. His numerous symptoms include prolonged jaundice (yellow skin); abnormalities in the structures of the cardio-vascular system, vertebrae of the spinal column, eyes, and kidneys; narrowing of the pulmonary arteries; characteristic facial features; shortened fingers; and stunted growth. The scarcity of bile ducts in his liver results in insufficient passage of bile to the small intestine, and malabsorption of fat-soluble vitamins and nutrients.

Joey's inability to grow, along with his severe difficulty eating and enjoying foods, were important factors that helped lead to his diagnosis. Every meal was a struggle for both of us. He often cried, vomited, and arched at mealtime. Once we received his diagnosis, we learned that, although he was getting a sufficient

amount of food for a typical child to gain weight, his body was starving. He was not able to absorb enough fat or vitamins from the food he was given.

The gastrostomy tube provided a means to supply the additional calories, fats and vitamins Joey desperately needed. Under the supervision of doctors and dietitians, our family started experimenting with many different formulas, looking for ones that not only would allow Joey to grow, but enable him to feel well during and after eating.

Nutrition as a Foundation

As a family, we believe in good nutrition as a foundation for health. My husband and I typically eat a well-balanced diet and we wanted to provide good nutrition for Joey. Initially, we pumped a series of different prescribed commercial formulas into our son. He continued to struggle with weight gain and growth.

We felt that Joey's health and emotional well being both could be better served by providing a more varied diet, and so we started investigating the idea of providing a homemade blended formula for him. At first the concept seemed a bit daunting. We had many concerns associated with changing Joey's diet that needed to be addressed. Proper nutrition, calorie counts, Joey's tolerance of a homemade formula, storage and preparation, as well as the increased work involved in producing the formula, were some of our biggest concerns.

However, the potential benefits we envisioned far outweighed any concerns we had. We saw a homemade formula as a possible way to improve both Joey's health and his quality of life. We also saw this as an opportunity to be more directly involved in our son's nutrition. As a family, the decision to move toward a homemade blended formula made sense. It provided us with a greater sense of unity regarding nutrition and more importantly, more rewarding family mealtimes.

Specific Dietary Requirements

The first step was to discuss the idea of a homemade formula with Joey's doctors and his feeding team,: several specialists, a dietitian and his occupational therapist. A great deal of care and planning was needed to take into consideration all the specific dietary requirements imposed by Joey's syndrome.

For example, foods high in vitamins A, D, E, and K were considered important additions to his homemade blended formula. These vitamins are closely monitored for Joey and he is often deficient in them due to malabsorption caused by his liver disease.

His inability to absorb most fats was another issue to consider. His diet needs to include fats that are more easily broken down by his digestive system. MCT (medium chain triglyceride) oil was identified as an easily digestible fat for Joey's specific needs.

Another concern was the amount of protein appropriate for him. Due to complications with his kidneys, his doctors did not favor a diet too high in protein.

Calories were another aspect to be considered in diet planning. Joey's poor growth and inability to gain weight necessitated a very high-calorie formula. But his severe gastroesophageal reflux dictated that the calorie content of the formula not be too high. Through prior experience, we knew that if the calorie content was too high, he would most likely vomit.

Joey also has a very slow-emptying stomach. His stomach takes approximately three times longer to empty than a typical child. This contributes to his already severe reflux and causes him to have even less desire or appetite for oral foods. Joey also must take many prescription medications that cause side effects such as nausea, constipation and decreased appetite.

Lastly, in thinking about a homemade blended diet, we wanted to add foods that were known to be good for his specific medical condition. For example, both ginger and papaya are known to aid with reflux. We wished to incorporate many natural, whole foods into his diet that would satisfy his very specific nutritional needs as well as aid in his growth and development.

In order to address all of these specific requirements, we needed our whole team to put their heads together to look at these issues in depth.

The good news was that by the time we knew enough to even ask about and discuss homemade blended food, Joey was three years old and his health status was relatively stable. Many of his doctors had a hard time understanding why I would want to work so hard when canned formula was so easy. Others were concerned that he wouldn't get adequate nutrition and calories. However, a few encouraged me and believed that there could be benefits from a more varied diet of fresh food that could not be obtained from a can.

Working with a dietitian familiar with Joey's dietary and health needs, we developed a plan to slowly start incorporating fresh foods into his blended diet. The first step was to calculate the calories per ounce required for his blended formula. Total daily calorie requirements as well as daily water requirements also were reviewed.

It was decided that the basis for Joey's homemade formula would be a predigested formula, Peptamen Junior®. This is formulated to be easier to digest than most formulas. It also contains MCT oil as its fat source. Joey had been successfully using this formula for several months. Using a well-tolerated formula as the base of our homemade formula gave us confidence that we could accurately detect any adverse reactions to new foods. It also helped relieve any anxieties about Joey receiving enough calories, vitamins and nutrients through the homemade formula. Starting with Peptamen Junior, we blended all new food additions directly into this base.

Set Goals

After all our research was complete and we had specific nutritional guidelines and a basic outline of a diet, we asked the doctors to review our plan and give their approval. Implementing the dietary changes, however, still required a great deal of care and planning. The team was called upon to investigate how to best introduce new foods into Joey's diet, and to set both short-term and long-term goals.

We set very small goals in the beginning. Each new introduction would be a baby food that we introduced very slowly. We felt that using baby food was a safe way to introduce a new food that was pure and quantifiable.

Our starting goal was to introduce one new food to Joey's diet every four days. Carrots were the first vegetable chosen because they're a good source of vitamin A, a vitamin in which Joey is deficient. The first day, a few spoonfuls of baby food carrots were blended with the Peptamen Junior and fed to Joey for just one meal. We watched closely for signs of intolerance to the carrots, such as increased reflux and vomiting, arching, and general crankiness.

When everything seemed to be going well, the next day we increased the number of meals that included blended carrots. At the end of the four day period, we were able to include carrots in three meals a day, and to substantially increase the amount of carrots. We felt confident that carrots were well tolerated and that we could move on to introducing another new food.

This methodology worked well for introducing new foods to Joey. We started with baby food fruits and vegetables before moving on to baby food meats. Fortunately, Joey tolerated new additions well and within a few months we had a basic homemade blended formula available to feed our son.

The formula contained the commercial canned formula base with added baby food fruits, vegetables, meats and cereals. The majority of

Joey's nutrition continued to be provided by the canned formula. We were very cautious about increasing the amount of homemade formula given.

We closely monitored Joey's growth during this initial phase of our plan and were encouraged by the results. He made small improvements in weight gain and continued to tolerate his homemade blended formula well. There were some setbacks to overcome, however.

Joey's very severe reflux and slow stomach emptying always have been a problem for him. At times his tummy troubles increase, especially if he's sick with a cold or flu. During these times, he tolerates the canned pre-digested formula better than his homemade blended formula. Sometimes we take a break from the homemade formula until he's feeling better; other times modifying the formula is necessary. When his reflux is at it's worst, a homemade formula that has fewer calories per ounce and is lighter in consistency is much easier for his body to accept.

We came to realize that making a homemade blended formula was not only a labor of love, but also an exercise in flexibility. It's a slow process that's always changing and evolving. We tried different foods and different amounts of the homemade formula based on Joey's health and stability at the time. We consulted with our team frequently to set new short term goals. Often we would set goals increasing the total amount of the homemade formula he received in a day. We also set goals of increasing the calorie content of his formula, with the hope of seeing additional weight gain. How and when these goals were met were totally dependent upon Joey and what was working for him at the time. We often felt that we took three steps forward, only to take two steps back.

The Next Step

We continued using baby foods for over a year, at which point he was able to tolerate approximately half of his nutrition from blended homemade formula. We saw dramatic improvement in his weight gain and growth, as well as improved overall health. We had met our short-term goals and were now ready to set our sights on the long-term goal of becoming less dependent on canned formula and to supply the majority of Joey's nutrition in the form of homemade blended formula.

After discussions with Joey's medical and nutritional team, we decided that it was time to start adding whole fresh foods to his homemade formula recipe and to phase out the use of baby foods. It was at this point that the real learning about nutritional options and what was best for Joey's specific medical condition really began.

We had a lot of questions to consider. First and foremost, could a diet of fresh foods, with a great deal of variety, improve his overall health? Our experience with the baby food had been very positive, so we believed that the answer to that question was a definite yes. If we saw improvement with the simple addition of baby foods, what else was possible? We wondered if a varied diet could help improve his digestive system. Would specific foods help with his reflux or slow stomach emptying? Could we offer foods that improved his fat absorption? Were there some high-calorie additives that could be used in his formula to help with his weight and growth?

It was at about this time that we discovered that Joey was slightly hypoglycemic. We had always noticed that he was extremely food dependent and became remarkably cranky if too much time passed between meals. We wondered if the expansion of his homemade blended formula could somehow help support this need. We also realized that we needed to investigate the timing of his meals to determine if they needed to be more strictly scheduled.

The more we learned, the more questions we had. We realized that we had to take on these issues one at a time and continue to be flexible with Joey's diet. We always let his responses to changes be our guide.

Every food choice that we added to his diet was carefully considered. Naturally, we incorporated fresh fruits and vegetables first, since these are more easily digested than meat. We used foods that we knew he could tolerate based on our experience with baby foods. Vegetables, fruits and grains high in fiber also were recommended to help regulate Joey's gastrointestinal system and counteract the side effect of constipation caused by medication.

We looked at the vitamin contents of the fruits and vegetables and concentrated on choosing a large variety for the maximum nutritional value. Throughout our process however, we tried to use foods high in vitamins A, D, E, and K, the vitamins in which Joey is deficient. Carrots, yams and broccoli are all vegetables high in vitamin A. Salmon, sardines, milk and eggs are foods rich in vitamin D. Nuts, seeds and whole grains are foods that are high in vitamin E. Lettuces and cabbages have a high vitamin K content.

After looking at some of the foods that were high in the vitamins that Joey needed, I became a bit apprehensive about possible allergic food reactions. I personally suffer from severe allergies including a few food allergies, and I was concerned that some of the foods we were considering could cause allergic reactions. To avoid complicating Joey's medical condition, we visited a pediatric allergist to have him tested. Luckily, he tested positive for only a few foods, notably shellfish and watermelon. Needless to say, we don't include these in his homemade blended formula.

Once we were confident Joey could tolerate a wide variety of whole fresh fruits and vegetables, it was time to start introducing whole grains. In order to add a variety of grains, I started to make congee to add to his formula. Congee is a traditional Chinese porridge that can be made from any whole grain that is slow cooked. I began rotating different grains into Joey's diet, such as whole grain rice, barleys and millets. All were cooked slowly with water in a slow cooker.

Meats and fats were the next addition. Because of Joey's kidney condition, his diet couldn't contain a large percentage of protein. We experimented with lots of different protein sources, which included slow-cooked beans, tofu, eggs, soy nut butter and lean meats. Fish and chicken gave him no difficulty at all, however, beef and peanut butter weren't tolerated well.

Foods lower in fat were much easier for him to digest, but an additional fat source was needed to satisfy his dietary requirements. We had been using MCT oil in both Joey's canned and homemade blended formulas. He tolerated it well and it was medically recommended due to his liver's inability to process other fats. Based on research done on his syndrome, we decided to stay on MCT oil, and not try other oils such as olive oil or flax seed oil.

We also wanted to boost the formula's calorie count and so looked at a wide variety of dietary supplements. We wanted one that would increase calories without adding too much protein or sugar. Ultracare for Kids® powder was ultimately chosen, not only to boost calories but to help round out Joey's daily intake of vitamins and minerals.

For Joey, vitamin levels are critical to his overall health. He's given a blood test every three months to check his levels of vitamins A, D, E, and K, as well as iron and zinc. He takes prescribed supplements for each of these vitamins and minerals. By supplying many of these vitamins in his homemade formula through fresh foods and nutritional additives, we've actually had a few instances of Joey's vitamin levels rising too high. It's taken careful work with his dietitian and physicians to adjust both his diet and prescribed vitamins to keep his levels constant and in the normal range. At present, Joey no longer requires prescribed vitamin A or vitamin D. The levels of both of these vitamins in Joey's system are maintained solely through his diet.

Another area of recipe adjustment was dairy content. Our basic homemade recipe contained a great deal of milk, yogurt, powdered milk and some cheese. Although his symptoms were better, Joey still suffered from severe reflux, slow stomach emptying, constipation and hypoglycemia. One of his physicians, a specialist in integrative medicine, suggested trying a dairy-free diet. This would cut the amount of difficult-to-digest fat and sugar in his diet. Joey had not shown any reaction to milk during allergy testing, but we wondered if he was having difficulty digesting the milk and milk products. We decided to give a dairy-free diet a try.

We substituted many soy products for the milk products in Joey's diet and immediately saw improvement in his digestive system. His vomiting episodes decreased and he was much less constipated. His stomach emptying also improved and in turn he was able to tolerate greater volumes of food and gain weight more quickly. We also saw some improvement in his hypoglycemic symptoms. While we still keep to a fairly strict meal schedule, Joey does not seem to suffer as much if a meal is a little late.

Continuing Research

As time has gone on, we've tried numerous variations on Joey's homemade blended recipe, and have continued to research nutritional options to further improve his health.

We've tried foods known to have stomach soothing properties, such as fresh ginger, papaya, chamomile tea and licorice, and observed digestive improvement with the addition of papaya and ginger. We also added foods high in omega-3 to help support Joey's compromised cardiovascular system, as well as other nutritional supplements to support his overall health.

We've learned about the value of a variety of spices that have antioxidant effects and health benefits, and include several in Joey's formula. As a family, we enjoy well-spiced foods; therefore it seemed only natural to spice Joey's meals as well. We chose our spices carefully and, as with all additions to Joey's diet, we tried one at a time.

Our recipe continues to evolve and change as we gain more knowledge and as Joey's needs change. We have not yet answered all of our initial questions about homemade formulas and our son's specific needs, and we continue to ask new questions as time goes on.

The Results

At present we've been using homemade formulas for six years. It's an evolving, ever-changing process that's based on Joey's health status and our experience. One constant that we've observed is that a varied diet rich in nutritious foods has improved our son's health. He has continued to gain weight and has a much improved digestive system. He's constipated much less often and his reflux, while still a problem, is fairly well under control.

At this point in time, he receives the majority of his nutrition from his homemade blended formula. We also include table foods in his formula. Many times what he doesn't finish at the table is blended up and used in his g-tube as a bolus-fed meal. Joey receives a wide variety of foods that would be extremely difficult to get a typical 8-year-old child to eat.

It can't be emphasized enough that incorporating new foods into the diet of a tube fed child is an individual process and each new food should be approached with caution. Only one new addition should be made at a time to screen for any possible negative reactions. This was critical to consider with Joey because of his sensitive system and complex dietary needs. Each child's tolerance to solid foods or calories per ounce will vary. For some children, the addition of a few jars of baby food blended with the canned formula may be enough of a dietary challenge. We've worked very closely with a dietitian throughout our whole process to be sure his nutritional needs continue to be met.

The results and pay-off have been phenomenal. The biggest improvements were almost immediate. Joey's weight gain and growth dramatically improved. His height and weight

had never registered on the growth charts. Within about six months of altering Joey's diet, he finally reached the 5th percentile. At present, Joey is solidly at 25th percentile for both height and weight.

Another immediate improvement was a new interest in oral foods. There was a direct correlation between the switch to homemade blended foods and Joey's willingness to try new food tastes and textures. And, his interest in meal preparation is much greater since the addition of our homemade blended formula.

Puzzle Pieces

During our homemade blended formula journey, we did a great deal of research to "perfect" Joey's diet and improve his quality of life. We consulted nutritionists, therapists, the Internet, and books on nutrition and herbs. I consult a few books regularly; however, I've found an amazing amount of information about nutrition on the Internet. Along the way, we found some other options for Joey's care sometimes considered outside the mainstream. We realized that his homemade formula was a large piece of a bigger puzzle.

One of the puzzle pieces that we explored was the addition of nutritional supplements to Joey's diet. As part of our ongoing research, we've added several supplements such as CoQ10, omega-3, SAM-e, zinc and a probiotic. His various physicians suggested each of these supplements at various times to address specific aspects of Joey's health. CoQ10 and omega-3 both are taken to support Joey's cardiovascular system. Omega-3 also has the added benefit of improving focus and concentration. SAM-e has been shown in studies to support liver health. Zinc is a mineral that's often deficient in Joey's system. It's also essential for focus and concentration and we give it to him as part of his diet only when his blood tests show that he's deficient.

The probiotic, which is a source of beneficial bacteria for the intestinal tract, is given to support Joey's digestive system. Due to his severe reflux,

Joey must take a prescription medication that blocks the production of acid in his stomach. While this reduces the chances of damage to his esophagus, it also kills much of the "good" bacteria in his system that's required for proper digestion. The probiotic is a source of "good" bacteria and acts as a partial replacement.

Before starting any of these supplements, we researched each one with the help of our integrative medicine specialist, and tried each one individually, in order to gauge Joey's tolerance and reaction to each new addition.

We've seen measurable improvement in our son's overall health and stamina. We believe that these supplements, along with the great improvements in Joey's diet, have directly contributed to these changes.

Other puzzle pieces that we've investigated have included some alternative therapies and medical interventions. Joey has required a great deal of therapy since birth. His obvious developmental delays were addressed through physical, speech and occupational therapy.

In addition, over the years Joey has had therapies such as Auditory Integration Training and Sensory Integration Therapy. Both of these therapies have addressed his over-sensitivity to the world around him, including sounds, sights, tastes, and textures. The changes we've witnessed have not only improved his ability to tolerate a wider variety of foods and oral experiences, they've also improved his quality of life. He's much more comfortable dealing with everyday sensory challenges. Prior to these therapies, a trip to a department store reduced him to tears. The flood of visual and auditory input was intolerable for him.

Another important piece of our puzzle was to work closely with physicians and specialists who looked at the big picture of Joey's health and happiness. Included in Joey's "team" are a physician specializing in integrative medicine and an osteopathic physician specializing in cranial sacral manipulation. Both of these specialists have contributed greatly to Joey's overall well being. The integrative medicine specialist has been invaluable in our decision to add nutritional supplements. He has recommended specific dietary changes, including foods higher in antioxidant and nutritional content. He's also been instrumental in helping us research other non-mainstream therapies and treatments and their potential benefit for our son.

Our osteopathic physician also has greatly improved our son's life. Prior to beginning cranial sacral treatments and osteopathic manipulation, Joey at 3 years of age, had never, ever, slept through the night. He was constantly irritable and crying, walked noticeably crooked, and often seemed to be in pain. After his first appointment with the osteopath, Joey slept through the night and has continued sleeping through the night ever since. He's a much happier and healthier boy as a direct result of these treatments.

As our journey with Joey continues, we continue to gain knowledge about nutrition and to investigate other therapies that may have some benefit for him. Most recently we've been investigating self-hypnosis, relaxation techniques, therapeutic yoga and acupuncture as ways to help our son cope with the stresses brought on by his medical condition. We're also hoping these techniques can help improve his digestion and possibly increase his appetite.

We firmly believe that all these puzzle pieces are fitting together to improve our son's overall health. We'll continue to study nutrition and supplements, listen to those around us with similar experiences, and investigate alternative therapies. Our son's care is ever changing and evolving. We'll continue to strive to give him every opportunity to have the best possible health, nutrition, and quality of life.

150

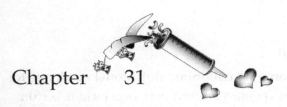

Chapter 31

Vegetarian Children
Marsha Dunn Klein, M.Ed., OTR/L

Many families follow a vegetarian diet and wonder if this can be offered to their tube fed child. It's possible to provide nutritious and varied vegetarian diets for orally fed children; therefore, it's possible to provide nutritious and varied vegetarian diets for tube fed children. The same principles apply.

The same special care should be taken to ensure the child receives the full array of nutrients necessary for healthy, consistent growth. In addition, the vegetarian diet needs to be consistent with special dietary considerations for each individual child.

For infants, breast milk or commercial infant formula is the appropriate diet; older infants would receive solid food in addition to the breast milk or infant formula. Goat, soy or rice milk should not be used in place of breast milk or commercial infant formula during the first year of life, as these do not contain the appropriate balance of nutrients for a growing infant.

Because diets without meats and dairy can potentially lead to deficiencies in certain vitamins and minerals if the diet is not well planned, it may be helpful to consult with a dietitian experienced in vegetarian diets for children.

Common Types of Vegetarian Diets

Lacto-ovo vegetarian
> Foods included: Grains, legumes, nuts, seeds, fruits, vegetables, dairy products and eggs
> Foods not included: Meats, poultry and fish

Lacto-vegetarian
> Foods included: Grains, legumes, nuts, seeds, fruits, vegetables and dairy products
> Foods not included: Meats, poultry, fish , eggs

Vegan vegetarian
> Foods included: Grains, legumes, nuts, seeds, fruits and vegetables
> Foods not included: Meat, poultry, fish, eggs, dairy products and honey. Foods with any amount of animal products such as casein or whey are usually avoided.

Some people consider themselves vegetarian even if they include fish and/or poultry in their diets.

There are several nutrients that require special attention in a child's vegetarian diet. These include calories to supply energy, protein, vitamin B12, vitamin D, iron, calcium and zinc.

Energy

Because vegetarian diets may have fewer calories than those including meats and dairy products, young children may have a difficult time obtaining adequate energy (or calories). This can be an even bigger challenge for the tube fed child who also has volume restrictions. In general, if the child is offered a varied and well balanced diet of a homemade blended formula and is growing well with good energy, there are probably enough calories.

The child's pediatrician or dietitian can help assess the child's growth pattern and determine whether the caloric intake is adequate. Careful inclusion of fats in the form of avocados, nuts and nut butters, olives, seeds and seed butters can provide additional energy in smaller volumes for tube fed children. Dried fruits also can be a very rich and concentrated calorie source.

Protein

Vegetarians easily can meet their protein and amino acid needs through a varied diet of protein-containing foods, as long as the caloric intake is adequate. Variety is the key.

151

To take in complete proteins, it's not necessary to strictly combine foods in the same meal to create a balance of amino acids, as was once believed. The current recommendation is to provide a mixture of varied proteins throughout the day to provide essential amino acids necessary for good health.

Rich sources of protein for vegetarians include legumes (beans), tofu and other soy products, nuts and nut butters, seeds, tempeh, milk and dairy products, eggs, amaranth and quinoa. Whole grains, greens, potatoes and corn add to the protein intake.

B12

Vitamin B12 is important for maintaining healthy nerve cells and red blood cells. It's also necessary to help make DNA, which is the genetic material found in all cells. B12 is naturally found in foods that come from animals including meat, fish, poultry, eggs, milk and milk products. The recommended intake for B12 is low, so a diet that contains dairy products or eggs can easily provide adequate B12.

Foods rich in B12 that can be easily included in a vegetarian diet include fortified breakfast cereals, nutritional yeast and fortified soymilk. Breast milk and commercial formulas also are good sources of B12.

Recommended Daily Allowance for Vitamin B12 *

Age	Micrograms per Day
1-3 years	0.9
4-8 years	1.2
9-13 years	1.8
14-18 years	2.4
19+ years	2.4

*Institute of Medicine. Food and Nutrition Board. Dietary Reference Intakes: Thiamin, riboflavin, niacin, vitamin B6, folate, vitamin B12, pantothenic acid, biotin and choline. National Academy Press. Washington, DC, 1998.

Iron

A common childhood nutritional challenge for both vegetarians and non-vegetarians is iron deficiency anemia. Rich sources of iron are whole and enriched grains and grain products, fortified baby foods and breakfast cereals, legumes, orange or dark green vegetables, egg yolks and blackstrap molasses. Iron absorption is enhanced by pairing foods rich in vitamin C and iron at the same meal.

Check with your child's pediatrician to see if your child is getting sufficient iron in the diet or if an iron supplement is indicated.

Calcium

Most people know that calcium is needed for strong bones and teeth. It's also necessary for nerve and muscle function and blood clotting. These tasks are a priority for a healthy body and if calcium from the diet is low, the body will use calcium from the bones for these other functions.

Calcium is found in foods such as fortified breakfast cereals, fortified soy milk, calcium fortified orange juice, tofu that is made with calcium sulfate, dairy products, dark green leafy vegetables such as collard greens, and blackstrap molasses.

Zinc

The best and most common food sources of the mineral zinc are meat and yogurt. Since these foods are often omitted from strict vegetarian diets, other foods sources of zinc should be added, such as whole grains and whole grain cereals, brown rice, legumes, hard cheeses, nuts, spinach, tofu and miso.

Vitamin D

This is found in fortified milk, egg yolks and fish—foods often omitted from a vegetarian diet. The body also makes vitamin D when exposed to sunlight. It requires 20-30 minutes of sun exposure on hands and face each day. Some children who live in sunny climates do not have a problem with vitamin D deficiency. For children who aren't regularly exposed to the sun, consider soy milk fortified with vitamin D, or discuss the use of a supplement with your child's pediatrician or dietitian.

Fiber

Diets of young children should not have excessive amounts of fiber, because this may decrease the amount of food they are comfortable eating and may inhibit the absorption of some nutrients. Giving the child some refined grain products and fruit juices can reduce the fiber content of a vegetarian child's diet.

By carefully following these guidelines, a vegetarian diet can be a healthy choice for a tube fed child receiving a homemade blended formula.

Recommended Daily Allowance of Fiber for Children

Age	Dietary Fiber
1-3 years	19 grams per day
4-8 years	25 grams per day
9-13 years, males	31 grams per day
14-18 years, males	38 grams per day
9-13 years, females	26 grams per day
14-18 years, females	26 grams per day

*Based on 2002, the Food and Nutrition Board of the National Academy of Sciences Research Council issued Dietary Reference Intakes (DRI) for fiber

For additional information see:

Jackson, P. (2006). *Vegetarian Baby and Child: Nutritional Guidance and Recipes to Help Raise a Healthy Child*. New York, NY: New Line Books.

Yntma, S.K., Beard, C.H. (1999) *New Vegetarian Baby*. Ithica, NY: McBooks Press.

Klein, M.D. and Morris, S.E. (2007). *Homemade Blended Formula Handbook.*
(Tucson, AZ: Mealtime Notions, LLC.)
Appendix C - Food Sources of Protein.
Appendix E - Food Sources of Fiber.
Appendix G - Food Source of Vitamin C.
Appendix J - Food Sources of Vitamin B12.
Appendix L - Food Sources of Iron.
Appendix O - Food Sources of Calcium.

USDA, Choose My Plate Vegetarian Resources
http://www.choosemyplate.gov/healthy-eating-tips/tips-for-vegetarian.html
http://www.choosemyplate.gov/food-groups/downloads/TenTips/DGTipsheet8HealthyEatingForVegetarians.pdf

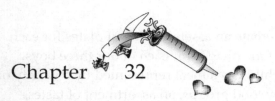

Chapter 32

Our Vegetarian Experience

Jenn Sandman

As I try to outline the progression my husband and I have taken with regards to our son Harper's blended food diet, I realize it is a constant work in progress.

We're constantly augmenting, readjusting and evolving Harper's diet as he grows and changes. The ability to adapt and be flexible is so important with tube fed children, just as it is for orally fed children.

But there are a few constants and commonalities. Above all, whatever we've chosen to feed Harper has been, at that point in time, the best answer for us as a family and for Harper as a child.

Harper was put on nasogastric tube feedings around the age of 8 months. He had been exclusively breastfed up until this point, but was diagnosed with failure to thrive from severe reflux and vomiting. He wouldn't try any foods except for nursing and severely restricted his time at the breast due to discomfort.

When the nasogastric feedings were started, and for their duration of three months, I felt very strongly that Harper should remain on a base of breast milk. In order to increase caloric density, I pumped milk throughout the day, mixed it with a supplement powder prescribed by Harper's gastroenterologist and dietitian to increase calories, and then my husband or I gave it to him as a bolus feeding with a syringe during the day, or by feeding pump at night. He also was encouraged to nurse on demand throughout the day and night. As a lactation counselor, I was very adamant about preserving our breastfeeding relationship, for a multitude of reasons.

At the age of 11 months, Harper clearly was not able to sustain weight via oral intake and received a gastrostomy tube. In a way, this time was exciting for us, as the diameter of the gastrostomy tube was greater than that of the nasogastric tube, so I could begin introducing pureed solids to him,

just as I had done with my other sons at the same age. Of course, we did so under the guidance, direction and approval of his pediatrician, dietician and gastroenterologist. Harper continued to nurse throughout the day and night.

In the beginning, I was fanatical about counting calories and measuring volumes, and was scrupulous about quantifying percentages from fats, carbohydrates and protein. We used commercial baby foods such as fruits, vegetables and grains and then added healthy oils to them to increase caloric density. Harper was getting as many as nine small meals a day because of the volume limitations imposed by his severe reflux. Everything was computed, checked and rechecked for the appropriate ratios.

Going Meatless

The amount of protein in Harper's food was always on the high side, based on his physical requirements. But we were struggling with inadequate weight gain and knew that as protein percentage increased, his propensity for weight gain was reduced. This is a similar principle as is found in the high-protein Atkins diet.

In an attempt to moderate the level of protein he was getting throughout the day, we began at an early point to omit meat from Harper's diet and monitor other sources of protein.

Different people define vegetarian diets in many ways. A vegan diet includes only food from non-animal sources. Other vegetarian diets exclude meat, but include milk, yogurt, cheese, other dairy foods and eggs. Harper's diet included dairy and eggs, but omitted meats.

When he became, in effect, a vegetarian, the differences in his overall health and weight gain were astounding. Although I'm a vegetarian (while my husband and two other sons are not vegetarian outside of our home), I wouldn't necessarily say that meat was detrimental to Harper. His diet without meat simply became better rounded, more proportional calorically, and, without a doubt, healthier for him.

Harper's protein requirements throughout the day were easily met by organic foods such as dairy, yogurt, egg, tofu, legumes and grains. In fact, his protein amounts are still at the top end for his recommended range! The fats he is getting tend to be healthier fats like flax seed oil, avocado, and olive oil.

We make sure to feed him a variety of grains (such as quinoa) that are naturally high in protein. Of course, he gets plenty of non-acidic fruits and vegetables. And we use a wide assortment of colors of vegetables, and provide adequate hydration with plenty of water.

An Evolving Diet

Although the vegetarian-based composition of Harper's blended food has been a constant for the past two years or so, the mindset behind his feedings has changed greatly.

In the beginning, of course, we were doing baby purees, even from a baby food jar, as the whole feeding thing was so new. After a number of months, as our confidence built, we began to prepare large batches of homemade pureed foods and freeze them in meal-size portions. I would prepare a vegetable batch, a fruit batch, a grain batch and a yogurt batch. Harper would get one of each throughout the day. I went through agony (calculator, pen and pencil, food scale, nutrition appendix, you name it) making sure that each recipe appropriately met his daily breakdown of requirements.

As Harper has recently celebrated his third birthday, his age and healthy weight have afforded us a bit more flexibility with regards to meal planning. What we do now is perfect for a healthy, just-weaned three year old, but wouldn't have felt safe two years ago for a child with a brand-new gastrostomy tube.

I now create an assembly line of plates for each meal. One plate is for each of our three boys. Each child has a meal represented by a variety of healthy food groups, an assortment of tastes, textures, vitamins and other nutrients.

All plates are composed of age-based portions. Harper's lunch plate, for example, is the exact plate you might feed any three year old vegetarian child. The meal might include hummus and whole-wheat pita points with olive oil drizzled on top, fresh strawberries, broccoli with ranch dressing and a glass of fortified vanilla soymilk. We all eat lunch together. The older boys usually eat most of their meal, and on a good day Harper will orally consume about a teaspoon of food from his plate. When the meal is over, I take his plate and dump it into the blender with the glass of soymilk and blend it into a smooth formula. As soon as it's blended, I feed him the meal through his feeding tube. It's so easy!

The same process is used for breakfast, lunch, and dinner, plus an extra snack before bedtime. Of course, we still do regular evaluations of his diet with a dietitian to make sure he's getting the appropriate nutrients, calories and foods. We make minute adjustments here or there as needed. For example, we might add more yogurt for calcium or increase the amount of fats containing omega-3. But on a whole, it's just like feeding any other vegetarian child.

In creating a homemade blended formula diet for a child, there are a number of attitudes and approaches that help parents move toward nutritious and happy meals. I feel the most important aspect is the ability to change with your child's needs and growth. What works today might not work tomorrow, or yesterday.

Be open-minded. Have a support system of professionals to ensure that your child is getting the best nutrition possible. And above all, remember that your child is just that — a child like any other! The same principles for preparing meals apply for every child.

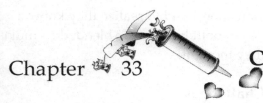

Chapter 33

Supporting Parents Who Choose a Homemade Blended Formula

Marsha Dunn Klein, M.Ed., OTR/L

It's one thing to decide that you want to provide a homemade blended formula for your child; it's quite another to know how to start! Parents in this position want and need support.

Because the movement to provide homemade blended foods by tube has been somewhat of a grassroots endeavor, often lead by parents rather than the medical community, families haven't been able to consistently find professionals with enough experience to answer all their questions. Support has had to come from health care providers with experience or who are willing to learn with the family, and from other parents providing homemade blended food to their children.

Each of these groups has used as a foundation the knowledge, guidelines and common sense used in feeding children who eat by mouth.

Medical Support

Because of the multiple medical challenges facing many tube fed children, it's best to discuss your interest in homemade blended formulas with your child's medical team.

Are there special dietary needs or restrictions dictated by your child's medical condition? Is there any medical reason why a homemade blended formula cannot be considered? What type of dietary transitions would your child's physician be recommending if your child could eat orally?

Dietitian Support

We encourage every family considering a homemade blended formula to discuss questions and their child's energy and growth needs with a pediatric dietitian.

Ideally, the dietitian will help families know where to start in the slow transition from a commercial formula toward a homemade blended

diet. The dietitian will monitor growth and nutritional needs and analyze homemade blended formula recipes as they evolve for each child. Nutritional needs change as children get older or as health and medication regimens change. Dietitians can provide essential support in these changes.

Parent Support Groups

Some locations have regular meetings of homemade blended formula groups. In these groups, parents and professionals share experiences and learn from each other. What works? What doesn't? What clogs the tube? What blenders work best? How do you keep the syringes working well?

Regular group meetings have been central for collecting and sharing information on this subject. We recommend the group include a dietitian, pediatrician and feeding therapist, not only to provide resource information, but also to learn from parents. Learning on this topic flows in both directions.

For example, one group met regularly to discuss what was working or not working for particular children and families. They discussed ups and downs of homemade blended formulas, and shared tips on recipes, presentation techniques and formula preparation. Each meeting also included a guest speaker who provided related information. Speakers were pediatricians, gastroenterologists, feeding therapists, dietitians, a Chinese herbologist, a cranial sacral doctor of osteopathy, and of course, parents with personal experience.

There also was a supply exchange in which families brought in extra supplies they no longer needed. And, since the discussions revolved around food issues, parents took turns bringing in the Vita-Mix high-powered blender to create tasty group snacks demonstrating the versatility of the blender to those new to the group.

Parent-to-Parent Support

Families with experience with homemade blended formulas often support parents just beginning the process. This support has taken the form of group meetings, as mentioned above, as well as formal and informal mentor programs. Some cities have a formal phone network. If a family wants to explore homemade blended formula nutrition, they're connected with a dietitian and a specific family who has had positive experiences they are willing to share.

Several informal Web-based support groups have evolved around the topics of tube feeding and homemade blended formulas. Veteran parents have graciously shared their experiences, positive and negative, and provided other parents with starting information and starting questions.

Professional Organizations

There are many resources for transitioning orally fed children from breast or bottle to solids: books, Internet sites, videos, handouts at pediatrician offices and guidelines through the American Dietetic Association and the American Academy of Pediatrics. There are entire shelves in bookstores and libraries devoted to this topic.

Though none of these sources focuses specifically on the transitions involved in tube feeding meals, many of the principles are the same. Just as you would make slow and gradual changes and follow the child's lead and responses when offering oral foods, you also must move slowly and follow the child's responses when offering a homemade blended formula to the child who is tube fed.

Just as you would add one new food and watch for allergies with each oral food, you must add one new food and watch for allergies with each new addition to the tube feeding formula. Essentially, parents are encouraged to use the solid information they already have about oral

food transitions, and to realize they know a great deal more about homemade blended formulas than they thought!

The Challenges

The challenge is to find professionals who believe in homemade blended formulas as an option for your tube fed child. Work with them. The challenge is to find professionals who have information about homemade blended formulas and the knowledge of how to make the transition from canned formula, or to find professionals willing to learn with you. Share with them.

The challenge is to remember that tube feedings are mealtimes too, and that you know quite a bit about feeding children. Enjoy the mealtime!

The challenge is to find informational, technical and emotional support as you move towards a homemade blended formula.

Quotable Quotes

How do I know you will be providing all the appropriate nutrients for your child with homemade blended formula?

Dietitian

How do you know I am providing all the appropriate nutrients for my other three children?

Parent

If I meet a child who is 18 months old who is only on breast milk or commercial formula, I am concerned. Why wouldn't I be concerned about a tube fed 18-month-old child who is only on breast milk or commercial formula?

Pediatritian

My tube fed eight year old gets better nutrition by tube than any child in his second-grade class! Their favorite foods are chicken nuggets, pasta, French fries and snack foods. My tube fed child gets an incredibly varied homemade blended diet including foods such as salmon, Brussels sprouts, beets, spinach, exotic grains, and liver, which none of his eight year old friends would eat.

Mother

For additional parent resources:

Food Selection & Recipes

Drink Your Meals	www.drinkyourmeals.com
Functional Formularies	http://functionalformularies.com
Just Food	www.justfood.org
Real Food Blends	www.realfoodblends.com

Foundations Supporting Feeding & Mealtimes

Nourish	www.nourishaz.org
Oley Foundation	http://www.oley.org

Internet Resources (Articles, Blogs, Books, Continuing Education Courses, & Feeding Products)

Blended Food Resource Group	www.foodbytube
Complete Tube Feeding: Everything you need to know about tubefeeding, tube nutrition and blended diets (Eric Aadhaar O'Gorman)	https://www.createspace.com/3811540
	www.mealtimenotions.com
	www.new-vis.com
Feeding Matters	www.feedingmatters.org
Feeding Tube Awareness Foundation	www.feedingtubeawareness.org
Mealtime Connections, LLC	http://www.mealtimeconnections.com
Mealtime Notions, LLC	http://www.mealtimenotions.com
New Visions	http://www.new-vis.com
You Start with a Tube	http://youstartwithatube.blogspot..com

For additional parent resources:

Listservs

Blenderized Diet Listserv   http://health.groups.yahoo.com/group/Blenderized-Diet

Feeding Listserv   http://health.groups.yahoo.com/group/feeding

G-Tube Listserv   http://listserv.syr.edu/scripts/wa.exe?SUBED1=gtube&A=1

Professional Organizations

Academy of Nutrition and Dietetics   http://www.eatright.org

Chapter 34

Commercial Formula Coverage

Marsha Dunn Klein, M.Ed., OTR/L

Parents of tube fed children and medical professionals aren't the only ones who have shown an interest in homemade blended formulas. Some third party payers, who cover the costs of commercial formulas for many tube fed children, are developing new policies that do not support children and their families. In some cases, they have gone so far as to abruptly terminate coverage for commercial formula, citing the homemade blended formula option as a justification. While we support efforts to reduce the skyrocketing costs of medical care, we cannot support such arbitrary decision-making.

Though we encourage homemade blended formulas when medically approved for tube fed children, we do not support policies that *require* it of families and preemptively terminate coverage for commercial formula, or policies that put decision-making at the third party payer level rather than in the hands of families and know-ledgeable professionals. Though extensive use of homemade blended formulas ultimately will reduce the costs of commercial formula for some families (and their third party payers), the cost savings will vary depending on each child's individual response.

The Decision to "Try"

When the decision is made to try a homemade blended formula, the emphasis is on ,try.` A family and medical team decide together that homemade blended formulas are a possibility. No parent or medical team member knows for sure if the transition to a homemade blended formula will work for that specific child. It's inappropriate to project or demand a date when the commercial formula will be discontinued. Many vital factors come into play. Neither the family, physician nor dietitian knows if the child can tolerate the dietary diversity, whether the child can take in adequate calories, or if the child will be able to grow adequately using a

homemade formula. Clearly, a third party payer would be even less able to make that decision.

Slow Food Introduction

Introducing food to tube fed children is a gradual process. Sometimes the child is given as little as half a teaspoon of a new food at a time. Very gradually, providing there is evidence of good gastrointestinal tolerance and growth, the homemade blended diet can move forward. However, there are many children who do not tolerate initial attempts to present blended foods. The process needs to be discontinued and tried again later, when the child's medical status improves. Moving forward too fast can aggravate gastrointestinal issues.

Sensitive Gastrointestinal Systems

Tube fed children often have sensitive or poorly functioning gastrointestinal systems. The very process of tube placement can interfere with normal gastrointestinal physiology. Introduction of homemade foods can help improve gastrointestinal challenges. For some children, bowel health, reflux and growth improve. For others, the gastrointestinal system is NOT ready. When the timing isn't right, the process needs to be stopped and tried again later.

"THE" Recipe

Some third party payers are demanding that dietitians provide ,THE` recipe for homemade blended food so commercial formula may be discontinued. ,THE` recipe does not exist. Each child has different caloric, protein, micronutrient and energy demands and a recipe right for one child isn't automatically right for another. There are guidelines for pureed recipes that then are modified based on the individual child's weight, energy needs, allergies, volume tolerances and family's cooking style, religious and cultural preferences. If the child tolerates a homemade blended formula and shows good growth, then the team knows they're on the right track for that child's recipe.

Volume Tolerance

Children who are tube fed are notoriously sensitive to volume changes. It's difficult to provide the same level of nutrients per ounce in homemade blended food as it is in a commercial formula. Often, to blend the food smoothly and thin enough to pass easily through the tube, more liquid must be added. This in turn increases the volume of food, making a complete transition to a blended formula impossible for some children.

Continuum

It's unrealistic to demand a completely homemade blended diet for all tube fed children. There is a continuum of options for modifying commercial formula diets. Some children only can tolerate one baby food fruit or vegetable being added to their commercial formula, once a day. Other children may have some purees mixed with the commercial formulas during daytime boluses and receive drip feedings of a commercial formula at night. Many children gradually tolerate expanded food choices until on a complete HBF diet, with the elimination of commercial formula. Some compliment their homemade blends with premade blended meals such as Real Food Blends. (www.realfoodblends.com)

Monitored Growth

For a multitude of reasons, children who are tube fed often have difficulty growing. Any change towards a blended food diet must include regular monitoring of growth. Growth MUST be appropriate. Cutting back the commercial formula too rapidly can stop a good growth pattern, putting the child at risk for malnutrition and failure to thrive.

Support

Some enthusiastic third party payers have abruptly cancelled commercial formula coverage without offering support to the family. Other families have been sent to a dietitian for consultation, only to discover that the dietitian has no experience helping children transition to a homemade blended formula. This is a new area for many medical personnel. They're often learning with the families. There must be a support system in place that covers all the necessary dietary and medical support before a child can begin the slow transition to a homemade blended formula.

Ultimately, if a family chooses to try a homemade blended formula and it works well for their child, the amount of commercial formula needed can be gradually decreased, as tolerance of blended purees increases. But because each child's response to a homemade blended formula is so different, families and medical teams, not third party payers, must be in charge of all decisions that relate to tube feeding diets.

In Summary

We support families and medical teams who are considering trying a homemade blended formula for a child. The decision to introduce some homemade foods into a diet is just a starting point. Because it's so unclear when, or if, the child will proceed, there should be no externally determined timelines for reducing commercial formula coverage. Commercial formulas will continue to be important dietary elements for some time during the transition, and may never will be completely discontinued. Families who decide to try a homemade blended formula need sufficient dietary, emotional and medical support from the beginning of their efforts, for proper knowledge and monitoring of this process. It's reasonable that third party payers want to reduce commercial formula costs, but because of the unique complexity of each tube fed child, third party payers should not be making decisions about discontinuing commercial formula. This decision needs to be made solely by a family with their medical team.

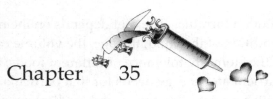

Frequently Asked Questions

Suzanne Evans Morris, Ph.D, CCC
Marsha Dunn Klein, M.Ed., OTR/L

Chapter   35

The Concept of a Homemade Blended Formula

What is a homemade blended formula?

We have defined homemade blended formula, or HBF, for the purposes of this book, as any formula that a parent makes to modify or replace a standard commercial formula with "real" foods. The "homemade" in the definition celebrates the personal nurturing nature of the preparation.

Why should I switch to a homemade blended formula?

There are no "shoulds" in the decision to make a homemade blended formula. We support it as an option to be considered with approval from your child's medical team. It is being used to provide dietary diversity for many tube fed children.

Why hasn't my doctor or dietitian advised me To give my child a homemade blended formula?

Many doctors and dietitians have had limited experiences with homemade blended formulas. There has been limited information available.

How do I know if a homemade blended formula is working for my child?

You know a homemade blended formula is working for your child just as you know a particular diet is working for any child. Your child will grow, and demonstrate optimum health. You will know it is working for you, as a parent, because you are feeling positive about the nutritional choices you are making and the time you spend in nourishing your child.

I do not have much time. Do I have to blend everything?

Absolutely not. Many families have successfully modified their child's diet by just adding some baby food to the child's diet. Remember that a homemade blended diet can be anything from formula or breast milk with a little baby food fruit or vegetable added to a completely pureed diet with no formula base.

It is so much easier to use commercial formula. Is it wrong if I want to just keep on doing what I am doing?

Commercial formulas have been providing nutrition for tube fed children for years. They are safe, convenient, readily available, and work for many families. We support family choice with medical support on this decision.

Are there some children who should not receive a homemade blended formula?

Some children have specific metabolic needs or severe and pervasive allergies that require highly specialized formulas. These children typically need a specialized medical formula and may not be candidates for a homemade blended formula.

Complete homemade blended diets are generally not considered for children who receive nasogastric tube feedings because of the small size of the tube and the significantly greater liquid content necessary for the blend to pass through the tube. Some families do a partial homemade blended formula diet (for example, by adding a diluted fruit or vegetable here or there), but most families wait until there is a gastrostomy tube for greater blended food concentrations.

Jejunal feedings that bypass the stomach and take food directly into the small intestine require special considerations by the medical team. Many dietitians and physicians prefer presentation of a predigested formula in the jejunum, but some are trying limited regular formula or blended diets. The jejunum is smaller than the stomach and lacks elasticity, so boluses and fast feedings are not recommended. See the detailed discussion of these specific issues in this book. Discuss the specific recommendations of your doctor and dietitian.

Making and Monitoring Formulas

What is the difference between a dietitian and a nutritionist?

Dietitians are required to have a minimum of a bachelor's degree in nutrition sciences or nutrition and dietetics from an accredited college or university. They must complete an accredited supervised practice program, and then pass a national certification examination and must maintain continuing educational requirements. The term, nutritionist, is used by many dietitians; however, it is more widely applied to individuals who do not have the professional credentials of a dietitian.

What is the difference between a homemade blended formula and pureed food?

A homemade blended formula is defined as any formula that a parent makes to modify or replace a standard commercial formula with "real" foods. The "homemade" in the definition celebrates the personal nurturing nature of the preparation. Purees are blended foods that can be offered orally or utilized as components of homemade blended diets.

Where do I start?

Check with your child's physician.

What equipment is needed to make a homemade blended formula?

Initially a standard inexpensive blender can be used to blend commercial formula and a small amount of baby food or a single puree. As recipes become more complex and more whole foods are used, a high powered blender, such as a Vita-mix or Blendtec, blends foods more efficiently and reduces the need to strain out lumps that can clog the feeding tube.

What is "The Recipe"?

There is not one particular recipe for a homemade

blended formula. The diet depends on the medical condition of the child, the age, the volume capacity of the stomach, tolerance of different foods, and nutrient and energy needs for that particular child. With support of dietitians and medical personnel, most families begin with one food at a time and add nutrients and calories as the child tolerates them until the puree offered becomes a well-balanced blend of foods.

In order to get in enough calories, the volume of food seems huge! How can I get my child to take all of it?

In order to get blended food into the tube, it must be in a thin enough and smooth enough state. Thinning the foods changes the caloric value so it is necessary to carefully look at the actual foods— the nutrients and calories received, not just the volume. There are creative ways to add calories with little volume. Some foods have more calories than others. The process of offering enough calories for growth needs to be a slow one so that the commercial formula is initially used as a base, providing sufficient calories and nutrients. As the child becomes accustomed to the formula and to taking larger amounts comfortably, foods are added gradually, observing the child's reaction and growth. The amount of the commercial formula may be reduced or eliminated over time.

How can I make sure my child is getting enough calories?

Watch your child's growth. Growth will be reflected in the growth chart. Children follow their own growth curve. Thus, a child who is at the fifth percentile may remain at that same percentile as he grows older and is taking in more calories. Initially dietitians monitor whether a child continues to grow at the same rate when a homemade blended formula is used.

How do I know my child is getting the required nutrients?

Work with your child's dietitian to analyze the homemade diet. Dietitians will help you understand the balance of nutrients and whether the current homemade blended formula recipe an needs modification.

How can I travel with a homemade blended formula?

You can travel with a homemade blended formula, but need to be very mindful about sanitary conditions to avoid contamination. See Chapter 22, Traveling with Homemade Blended Formulas, for suggestions.

What is the shelf life of a homemade blended formula? Can it be frozen?

Homemade blended foods can be frozen as can homemade baby food. It is recommended that the individual food be used within a month and that the separate foods be combined with fluids and non-freezable ingredients at the time of serving.

How much additional water should I give my child?

Some families prime the tummy with a comfortable bolus drink of water 20-30 minutes before the bolus feeding. Remember, of course, that the amount of water needed by the child depends on the child's medical condition, activity level, and climate of residence. See Chapter 16, Homemade Blended Formulas and Hydration, for further suggestions.

What is the cost difference between a commercial formula and a homemade blended formula?

The cost of a homemade blended formula depends on if it is a complete homemade blended formula or if it is based on a commercial formula. And it depends on whether the homemade blended formula has a small amount of puree added, or whether it is mostly puree. Within the group of families making purees there is a continuum from buying commercial baby food for additions to cooking and preparing all purees from special organic farms and health food stores. All these variables influence the costs of the homemade blended formulas.

Equipment

What size tube works best?

Parents who are using a homemade blended formula with their children tell us they have had the easiest time offering homemade blended formulas when they use a 14 French diameter catheter or larger. Most families using button type tubes have success when using a bolus size extension (rather than the pump tubing) because it allows the thicker homemade blended formula to be presented. However, the "French" measurement (Ex. 14 Fr, 16 Fr, 18 Fr.) is the size of the tubing as it goes through the child's abdomen, but the inner workings of each feeding button is the same size, so there seems to be no difference in presentation of a homemade blended formula, from the tube perspective, with differing button French sizes. Of course, technology is changing and it will be important as newer tubes are designed and put into the market, to look at the tube of each child and determine how it works in relation to consistencies and volumes.

Can you put a homemade blended formula into a nasogastric tube?

Commonly, most gastrostomy tubes start at a diameter size of a 14 French or greater. Most nasogastric tubes for infants and young children are much smaller to allow for ease of placement in the narrow nasal passages. They are usually sized at about a 5 to 8 French; thus they are much smaller than a gastrostomy button or catheter tube. A homemade blended formula is more of a challenge, in general because it is thicker and can clog the tube if it is not pureed or thinned sufficiently. Options are considerably limited with nasogastric tube sizes.

Having said that, we know of parents who have successfully mixed single fruits and vegetables into the formula and provided it slowly through the tube to offer variation to the formula diet. The formula, however, remains predominantly the commercial formula in order to provide nutrients and calories in a reasonable volume and time.

Can you put a homemade blended formula into a jejeunal tube?

You must ask your child's doctor and dietitian. This generally has not been recommended or is cautiously recommended because the jejeunum, or top part of the small intestine is a digestive tube that is not intended to stretch and respond to the size of a meal or a bolus as a stomach does. Additionally, food placed directly into the top of the small intestine has not had the benefits of mouth digestion and the complex process of digestion that takes place in the stomach. Formulas generally recommended for direct jejeunal placement are specially prepared to be more broken down and more easily digested than regular infant and toddler formulas or than pureed foods.

Some dietitians, however, have had experience with some children with some homemade blended food in the jejunum. This <u>must</u> be checked out with your child's team as it is not approved for all children. Children often require jejeunal feedings in order to bypass the stomach to reduce the chronic cycle of vomiting and poor weight gain. Many of these children have gastrojejeunal tube combinations. Most physicians have encouraged the family to use the jejeunal tube as prescribed with special formula first. As the child's cycle of vomiting is reduced, some families have had success introducing very small quantities of easy to digest purees directly into the stomach, gradually increasing the volume as the child shows tolerance. Discuss options with your child's gastroenterologist.

How does a homemade blended formula affect the life of my child's feeding button?

Parents describe broad ranges of life for their child's feeding tubes and buttons, with and without homemade blended formulas.

Can I use a homemade blended formula with a feeding pump?

There are two considerations with the feeding pump. First of all, the thickened homemade blended formula can easily clog the pump and not flow well through the long tubing. A homemade blended formula can be used, but usually it is very diluted and is more formula-based than food-based. Secondly, there is an issue of food contamination when food sits out at room temperature too long. It is generally recommended that a homemade blended formula be delivered in less than two hours if it is given through a feeding pump. Chilling the food bag is recommended.

How do I move the puree through the feeding tube?

Most families prefer using the bolus extension tube because it has a larger diameter, and the thicker puree seems to move more easily through it. Syringe feeding provides the pressure needed to move thicker foods down the tube.

Supporting the Body

Can a homemade blended formula help my child's constipation?

Orally fed children benefit from increasing the amount of water, fruits, vegetables and fiber in the diet. Adding these components to the homemade blended formula can also help constipation for tube fed children.

Is a homemade blended formula safe if my child has medical problems?

Ask your child's doctors.

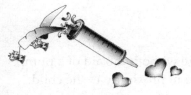

Appendix A — Tube Feeding Glossary

Bolus	A meal of homemade or commercial formula provided by tube in two hours or less.
Bolus Extension Tube	A piece of tubing that attaches a gastronomy tube to the syringe.
Bolus Meal	Another name for a bolus. A meal of homemade or commercial formula provided by tube in two hours or less.
Button	A small one-way valve device that is small and flush to the skin. A feeding tube is inserted into the button for meals and removed between meals.
Catheter	A type of feeding tube that extends from the abdomen.
Commercial Baby Food	The baby food available on the shelves and freezers of grocery stores that provides a variety of basic food nutrients for stages of infant eating. Various stages of complexity in food variety and textures are available to meet the emerging skills of infants and toddlers.
Commercial Formula	The canned, boxed or bottled formulas containing essential nutrients available for infants, toddlers and older children.
Congee	A grain cereal cooked slowly to preserve all of the nutrients.
Dietary Diversity	The concept of offering a varied diet in order to provide optimum nutrition.
Drip Feedings	Tube feedings offered from a feeding bag via pump or gravity.
Extensions	A plastic tube connecting the gastrostomy feeding button and the food source.
Feeder Diversity	Change in the person who presents the tube feeding.
Flow Rate	The speed at which the tube feeding is presented.
"French" Number Designation	"French" (Fr) is the tube diameter designated by a number and the letters "Fr". The bigger the number, the larger the diameter. (i.e., 14 Fr, 16 Fr)
G-J Tube	Gastro-jejeunal tube. This tube provides the option of giving tube feedings directly into the stomach or into the jejeunum.
Gastroesophageal Reflux	Contents from the stomach move out of the stomach into the esophagus or mouth. It is a problem for children when it causes discomfort, pain, appetite suppression, respiratory impairment, swallowing dysfunction, and decreased growth.
Gastrostomy Tube	G-Tube. The feeding tube goes directly through the abdomen into the stomach.

(Continued on next page)

Gravity Feeding	Tube feeding offered from a bag or syringe without the aid of a pump. The flow rate depends how high it is hung in proximity to the child.
HBF	An abbreviation for Homemade Blended Formula.
Homemade Blended Formula	A homemade blended formula, for the purposes of this book, is any formula that a parent makes to modify or replace a standard commercial formula with "real" foods. The "homemade" in the definition celebrates the personal nurturing nature of the preparation.
Jejeunal Tube	The jejunum is the part of the small intestine that lies between the duodenum and ileum sections. The jejeunal tube is a type of feeding tube that passes through the stomach and into the jejunum. It is most commonly used when children have severe reflux and vomiting or are unable to empty food from the stomach.
Mealtime Duration	The mealtime duration is the time needed to eat a meal orally or present a meal by feeding tube.
Mealtime Partners	People with whom you share a meal
Place Diversity	Different places where meals are shared.
Plunger	The part of the syringe that is used to push food or formula through the tip and into the feeding tube extension.
Pump Feedings	Tube feedings provided by a feeding pump, which allows the feeder to preset the rate and duration of formula flow.
Purpose Diversity	The different reasons we share meals; for example, for nutrition, celebration and social interactions.
Real Foods	Described, for the purposes of this book, as any foods that are used to make homemade formula, as contrasted with a commercial tube feeding formula.
Syringe	A small hollow cylinder used for presenting or withdrawing liquids or foods.
Tasting Bolus	Foods given to the tube fed child for oral tasting.
Venting	A procedure to help an infant or child release air or gas from the stomach. This is used primarily when a child has a fundoplication and is unable to burp.
Volume Tolerance	The amount of food or liquid the child handles comfortably at a specific meal or during an entire day.

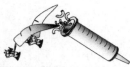 **Appendix B—Calorie Chart**

Grains	Quantity	Calories
Amaranth flakes	½ cup	67
Barley, cooked	½ cup	97
Buckwheat	½ cup	77
Bulgur, cracked wheat	½ cup	75
Couscous, cooked	½ cup	85
Cream of wheat, instant, prepared	½ cup	77
Millet, cooked	½ cup	104
Oatmeal, cooked with water	½ cup	74
Quinoa, cooked	½ cup	170
Rice, brown, cooked	½ cup	108
Rice, white, cooked	½ cup	102
Rice, wild, cooked	½ cup	82

Vegetables	Quantity	Calories
Alfalfa sprouts	½ cup	5
Artichoke hearts	½ cup	42
Asparagus	½ cup	22
Avocado	½ cup	120
Bamboo shoots	½ cup	12
Bean sprouts, canned	½ cup	5
Beans, green	½ cup	17
Beans, wax, cooked	½ cup	22
Beets, cooked	½ cup	29
Beet greens, cooked	½ cup	19
Bell pepper, fresh	½ cup	14
Bell pepper, boiled	½ cup	19
Broccoli, cooked	½ cup	22
Broccoli, fresh	½ cup	15
Brussels sprouts	½ cup	30
Cabbage, boiled, shredded	½ cup	17
Cabbage, fresh, shredded	½ cup	9
Carrots, fresh	½ cup	25
Carrots, sliced, boiled	½ cup	35
Cauliflower, boiled	½ cup	14
Cauliflower, fresh	½ cup	13
Celery, cooked, diced	½ cup	14

(Continued next page)

Appendix B—Calorie Chart (Continued from previous page)

Vegetables	Quantity	Calories
Chard, boiled	½ cup	18
Chard, fresh	½ cup	3
Chayote, boiled	½ cup	19
Collards, boiled	½ cup	25
Collards, fresh	½ cup	5
Corn, boiled	½ cup	76
Corn, creamed	½ cup	40
Eggplant, boiled	½ cup	13
Eggplant, fresh	½ cup	11
Fennel, fresh	½ cup	13
Kale	½ cup	17
Kohlrabi	½ cup	24
Leeks, chopped, boiled	½ cup	16
Mushrooms, fresh	½ cup	9
Mustard greens, boiled	½ cup	10
Nopales, cooked	½ cup	11
Okra, boiled	½ cup	30
Onion, chopped fresh	½ cup	34
Parsnips, boiled	½ cup	63
Peas, green, fresh	½ cup	52
Peas, snow, fresh	½ cup	13
Peas, snow, boiled	½ cup	34
Pepper, sweet, green, chopped, raw	½ cup	15
Pepper, sweet, red, chopped, raw	½ cup	20
Plantain, sliced, cooked	½ cup	90
Poi	½ cup	134
Potato, white with skin, boiled	½ cup	68
Potato, sweet, baked or boiled	½ cup	68
Pumpkin, boiled	½ cup	24
Radish, fresh	½ cup	9
Rutabaga, boiled	½ cup	33
Spinach, fresh	½ cup	4
Spinach, boiled	½ cup	21

(Continued next page)

Fruits	Quantity	Calories
Apple with skin	½ cup	32
Apple, dried	½ cup	72
Applesauce, sweetened	½ cup	97
Applesauce, unsweetened	½ cup	52
Apricots, canned in juice	½ cup	58
Apricots, canned in heavy syrup, drained	½ cup	92
Apricots, canned in light syrup, drained	½ cup	79
Apricots, dried	½ cup	105
Apricots, fresh	½ cup	39
Banana, sliced	½ cup	67
Banana, mashed	½ cup	100
Blackberries, fresh	½ cup	31
Blackberries, frozen, unsweetened	½ cup	48
Blueberries, fresh	½ cup	35
Blueberries, frozen, unsweetened	½ cup	40
Cantaloupe	½ cup	27
Casaba melon	½ cup	24
Cherimoya	½ cup	57
Cherries, sour, canned	½ cup	44
Cherries, sour, fresh, without pits	½ cup	39
Cherries, sour, frozen	½ cup	36
Cherries, sweet, canned	½ cup	57
Cherries, sweet, fresh	½ cup	46
Cherries, sweet, frozen, sweetened	½ cup	115
Cranberries, dried, sweetened	½ cup	187
Cranberries, fresh	½ cup	24
Dates, chopped	½ cup	126
Figs, dried	½ cup	185
Fruit cocktail, canned in juice	½ cup	57
Fruit cocktail, canned in heavy syrup	½ cup	93
Fruit cocktail, canned in water	½ cup	39
Gooseberries, fresh	½ cup	33
Grapefruit	½ cup	37
Grapes	½ cup	30
Guava, raw	½ cup	42
Honeydew melon	½ cup	32
Kiwi fruit	½ cup	54

(Continued next page)

Appendix B—Calorie Chart (Continued from previous page)

Fruits	Quantity	Calories
Mandarin oranges, canned in juice	½ cup	46
Mandarin oranges, canned in light syrup	½ cup	77
Mango	½ cup	54
Mincemeat	½ cup	180
Nectarine	½ cup	30
Orange	½ cup	42
Papaya	½ cup	27
Passion fruit	½ cup	114
Peaches, canned in heavy syrup	½ cup	95
Peaches, canned in juice	½ cup	54
Peaches, canned in light syrup	½ cup	68
Peaches, fresh	½ cup	33
Peaches, frozen, sliced	½ cup	25
Pear, canned in juice	½ cup	62
Pear, canned in heavy syrup	½ cup	94
Pear, canned in light syrup	½ cup	72
Pear, dried	½ cup	236
Pear, fresh	½ cup	48
Pineapple, canned in juice	½ cup	75
Pineapple, fresh	½ cup	38
Plum	½ cup	38
Plum, dried (prunes)	½ cup	204
Prickly pear fruit	½ cup	30
Prunes, dried	½ cup	204
Raisins	½ cup	109
Raspberries, frozen	½ cup	35
Raspberries, raw	½ cup	18-32
Rhubarb, cooked with sugar	½ cup	139
Rhubarb, fresh	½ cup	13
Strawberries, fresh	½ cup	22
Strawberries, frozen, sliced, sweetened	½ cup	61
Strawberries, frozen, unsweetened	½ cup	26
Tangerine	½ cup	43
Watermelon	½ cup	25

(Continued next page)

Appendix B—Calorie Chart (Continued from previous page)

Juices and Necters	Quantity	Calories
Apple juice	½ cup	58
Apricot nectar	½ cup	70
Carrot juice	½ cup	49
Grape juice	½ cup	75
Grapefruit juice	½ cup	51
Orange juice	½ cup	56
Papaya nectar	½ cup	70
Pear nectar	½ cup	70
Pineapple juice	½ cup	70
Prune juice	½ cup	90
Tomato juice	½ cup	21
Tomato/clam juice	½ cup	58

Milk and Dairy *In One-Cup Equivalents*	Quantity	Calories
Buttermilk, low fat	1 cup	98
Cheese, American	2 oz	212
Cheese, cheddar	1.5 oz	171
Cheese, cheddar, shredded	⅓ cup	150
Cheese, Colby	1.5 oz	168
Cheese, feta	1.5 oz	112
Cheese, mozzarella	1.5 oz	108 – 120
Cheese, mozzarella, shredded	⅓ cup	80-105
Cheese, Parmesan, shredded	⅓ cup	109
Cheese, Swiss	1.5 oz	162
Cheese, Velveeta	2 oz	170
Cottage cheese, creamed	2 cups	432
Milk, 1 %	1 cup	100
Milk, 2 %	1 cup	120
Milk, almond	1 cup	70
Milk, evaporated, whole milk	1 cup	300-400
Milk, goat	1 cup	168
Milk, rice	1 cup	120
Milk, skim	1 cup	85
Milk, soy	1 cup	80-120
Milk, whole	1 cup	150
Ricotta, part skim	½ cup	170
Ricotta, whole milk	½ cup	214
Yogurt, fruit, low fat	1 cup	244 – 260
Yogurt, plain, — whole milk	1 cup	150

(Continued next page)

173

Appendix B—Calorie Chart (Continued from previous page)

Meats	Quantity	Calories
Bacon, cooked	1 slice	40
Beef, bottom round	1 oz	52
Beef, ground, 85% lean	1 oz	71
Chicken, breast, cooked	1 oz	47
Chicken, leg, cooked	1 oz	54
Ham, roasted	1 oz	52
Lamb, roasted	1 oz	52
Liver, beef, cooked	1 oz	50
Pork loin, chops, broiled	1 oz	91
Pork tenderloin, roasted	1 oz	50
Pork loin, roasted	1 oz	66
Turkey, breast, cooked	1 oz	38
Turkey, ground, cooked	1 oz	67
Turkey, leg, cooked	1 oz	45

Fish	Quantity	Calories
Cod, broiled	1 oz	30
Halibut, broiled	1 oz	40
Herring, cooked	1 oz	58
Perch, broiled	1 oz	34
Salmon, fresh, broiled	1 oz	45-60
Salmon, canned	1 oz	30-40
Sardines, Atlantic, in oil, drained	1 oz	59
Sword fish, broiled	1 oz	50
Tuna, canned in oil	1 oz	55
Tuna, canned in water	1 oz	30
Tuna, fresh, broiled	1 oz	52

(Continued next page)

Appendix B — Calorie Chart (Continued from previous page)

Legumes	Quantity	Calories
Baked beans, canned with franks	¼ cup	92
Black beans, boiled	¼ cup	57
Fava beans, boiled	¼ cup	47
Garbanzo beans (chick peas), boiled	¼ cup	68
Hummus	2 Tbsp	55
Blackeyed peas, boiled	¼ cup	50
Great Northern beans, boiled	¼ cup	52
Kidney beans, boiled	¼ cup	55
Lentils, boiled	¼ cup	58
Lentil soup	½ cup	70
Lima beans, boiled	¼ cup	58
Navy beans, boiled	¼ cup	64
Navy bean soup	½ cup	70
Pinto beans, boiled	¼ cup	61
Red beans, boiled	¼ cup	55
Refried beans, canned	¼ cup	60
Soybeans, green (edamame)	¼ cup	64
Split peas, boiled	¼ cup	58
Split pea soup	½ cup	60
White beans, boiled	¼ cup	64

Oils/Fats	Quantity	Calories
Butter	1 Tbsp	102
Canola oil	1 Tbsp	120
Corn oil	1 Tbsp	120
Flax oil	1 Tbsp	120
Margarine	1 Tbsp	102
Olive oil	1 Tbsp	120
Peanut oil	1 Tbsp	119
Safflower oil	1 Tbsp	120
Sesame oil	1 Tbsp	120
Vegetable oil	1 Tbsp	120

(Continued next page)

Nuts, Nut Butters & Seeds	Quantity	Calories
Almond butter	1 Tbsp	101
Almond paste	1 Tbsp	65
Almonds, dry	½ oz	84
Brazil nuts	½ oz	93
Cashews, dry	½ oz	81
Cashew butter	1 Tbsp	94
Flax meal	1 Tbsp	37
Flax seeds	1 Tbsp	64
Macadamia nut butter	1 Tbsp	115
Macadamia nuts	½ oz	102
Peanut butter	1 Tbsp	100
Peanuts	½ oz	83
Pistachios	24	84
Pumpkin seed kernels	½ oz	77
Sesame butter (Tahini)	1 Tbsp	89
Sesame seeds	1 Tbsp	51
Sunflower seed butter	1 Tbsp	93
Sunflower seed kernels	½ oz	81
Walnut halves	7	46

Extras	Quantity	Calories
Avocado	½ medium	160
Avocado, cubed	½ cup	120
Condensed milk, sweetened, canned	1 Tbsp	75
Cream cheese	2 Tbsp	101
Dark corn syrup	1 Tbsp	57
Grape juice, frozen concentrate, sweetened, undiluted	1 Tbsp	33
Grapefruit juice, frozen conc. unsweetened, undiluted	1 Tbsp	25
Molasses, blackstrap	1 Tbsp	47
Orange juice, frozen conc., unsweetened, undiluted	1 Tbsp	28
Sorghum - sweet syrup	2 Tbsp	62
Wheat germ	2 Tbsp	51

Sources: Nutritionist Pro™ Nutrition Analysis Software from Axxya Systems www.nutritionistpro.com
(used with permission) and USDA Dietary Guidelines for Americans 2005 at www.health.gov/dietaryguidelines/

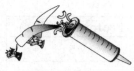

Appendix C - Food Sources of Protein

Meats	Quantity	Protein (Grams)
Beef, bottom round, cooked	1 oz	8 g
Beef, ground, 85% lean, cooked	1 oz	7 g
Chicken breast, cooked	1 oz	8.5-9 g
Chicken leg, cooked	1 oz	7.5 g
Ham, roasted	1 oz	6 g
Lamb, roasted	1 oz	7 g
Liver, beef, braised	1 oz	8 g
Pork loin, roasted	1 oz	8 g
Pork loin chops, broiled	1 oz	7 g
Pork tenderloin, roasted	1 oz	9 g
Turkey breast, cooked	1 oz	8 g
Turkey leg, cooked	1 oz	8 g
Turkey ground, cooked	1 oz	8 g
Veal, ground, broiled	1 oz	7 g
Fish	**Quantity**	**Protein** (Grams)
Crabmeat, steamed	1 oz	5 g
Crabmeat, imitation	1 oz	3.5 g
Halibut, cooked	1 oz	7.5 g
Lobster, cooked	1 oz	6 g
Salmon, fresh, poached	1 oz	6.5 g
Salmon, pink, canned, drained	1 oz	4 g
Scallops, steamed	1 oz	4.5 g
Shrimp, cooked	1 oz	6 g
Tuna, canned in oil, drained	1 oz	8 g
Tuna, fresh, cooked	1 oz	8 g
Tuna, light, canned in water, drained	1 oz	7 g
Dairy and Eggs	**Quantity**	**Protein** (Grams)
Cheese, American	1 oz	6 g
Cheese, cheddar	1 oz	7 g
Cheese, Colby	1 oz	7 g
Cheese, cottage, creamed	½ cup	13 g
Cheese, cream, regular	2 Tbsp	2 g
Cheese, feta	1 oz	4 g
Cheese, Monterrey Jack	1 oz	7 g
Cheese, mozzarella	1 oz	6-7 g
Cheese, Parmesan, grated	1 Tbsp	2 g
Cheese, ricotta, whole milk	½ cup	14 g

(Continued on next page)

Appendix C—Food Sources of Protein (Continued from previous page)

Dairy and Eggs	Quantity	Protein (Grams)
Cheese, Swiss	1 oz	7.5 g
Cheese sauce	¼ cup	6 g
Egg, white	1	3.5 g
Egg, yolk	1	2.5 g
Egg, whole, medium	1	6 g
Milk, 1%	1 cup	8 g
Milk, 2%	1 cup	8 g
Milk, almond	1 cup	2 g
Milk, coconut, canned	1 cup	5 g
Milk, evaporated whole milk, canned	½ cup	8.5 g
Milk, goat	1 cup	9 g
Milk, nonfat, dry, powder	1 Tbsp	2.5 g
Milk, nonfat, dry, prepared	1 cup	8 g
Milk, rice	1 cup	1 g
Milk, skim	1 cup	8 g
Milk, soy	1 cup	7 g
Milk, sweetened, condensed	1 Tbsp	½ g
Milk, whole	1 cup	8 g
Yogurt, plain	1 cup	7-13 g
Yogurt, soy	1 cup	5 g

Nuts and Seeds	Quantity	Protein (Grams)
Almond butter	1 Tbsp	2 g
Almond paste	1 Tbsp	1 g
Almonds, blanched	¼ cup	8 g
Almonds, dry roasted	¼ cup	8 g
Brazil nuts	¼ cup	5 g
Cashew butter	1 Tbsp	3 g
Cashews, dry roasted	¼ cup	5 g
Flax seeds	1 Tbsp	2 g
Flaxseed meal	1 Tbsp	1.5 g
Hazelnuts	¼ cup	5 g
Macadamia nut butter	1 Tbsp	1.5 g
Macadamia nuts, oil roasted	1 Tbsp	3 g
Peanut butter	1 Tbsp	4-4.5 g
Pecans	¼ cup	2.5 g
Pistachios	¼ cup	6.5 g
Sesame butter (Tahini)	1 Tbsp	2.5 g
Sesame seeds	1 Tbsp	1.5 g
Sunflower seed butter	1 Tbsp	3 g
Sunflower seeds, dry roasted	1 Tbsp	1.5 g
Walnut, pieces	¼ cup	4.5 g

(Continued on next page)

Appendix C—Food Sources of Protein (Continued from previous page)

Beans and Legumes	Quantity	Protein (Grams)
Baked beans, canned, with franks	½ cup	7 g
Baked beans, with pork	½ cup	6.5 g
Baked beans, canned, vegetarian	½ cup	6 g
Black beans, boiled	½ cup	8 g
Black-eyed peas, boiled	½ cup	7 g
Chickpeas (garbanzo beans)	½ cup	7 g
Edamame, boiled (green soybeans)	½ cup	11 g
Fava beans, boiled	½ cup	6 g
Great Northern beans, boiled	½ cup	7 g
Hummus	½ cup	3 g
Kidney beans, boiled	½ cup	8 g
Lentils, boiled	½ cup	9 g
Lima beans, baby, boiled	½ cup	7 g
Navy beans, boiled	½ cup	7 g
Pinto beans, boiled	½ cup	8 g
Red beans, boiled	½ cup	8 g
Refried beans, canned	½ cup	7 g
Soybeans, green, cooked	½ cup	11 g
Split peas, boiled	½ cup	8 g
Tofu	½ cup	2-3.5 g
White beans, boiled	½ cup	8 g
Grains	**Quantity**	**Protein (Grams)**
Amaranth, dry	½ cup	7 g
Amaranth flakes	½ cup	3 g
Barley, pearled, cooked	½ cup	2 g
Bread, white	1 slice	2 g
Bread, whole wheat	1 slice	3.5 g
Bread crumbs	¼ cup	1-4 g
Buckwheat	½ cup	3 g
Bulgur (cracked wheat)	½ cup	3 g
Corn tortilla	1	2 g
Cornmeal, whole grain, dry	¼ cup	2 g
Couscous, cooked	½ cup	3 g
Cream of wheat, instant prepared	½ cup	2 g
Millet, cooked	½ cup	4 g
Oats, old-fashioned, dry	½ cup	5 g

(Continued on next page)

Appendix C—Food Sources of Protein (Continued from previous page)

Grains	Quantity	Protein (Grams)
Oats, steel-cut, dry	¼ cup	6 g
Quinoa, dry	¼ cup	5.5 g
Rice, brown, cooked	½ cup	2.5 g
Rice, white, cooked	½ cup	2 g
Rice, wild, cooked	½ cup	3 g
Rye flour, whole	1 Tbsp	1 g
Sorghum	2 Tbsp	2.5 g
Wheat flour, whole	1 Tbsp	1 g
Vegetables	**Quantity**	**Protein (Grams)**
Broccoli, or cauliflower, cooked	½ cup	2 g
Broccoli, or cauliflower, raw	½ cup	1 g
Corn, cooked	½ cup	2.5 g
Greens, (kale, turnip, etc.)	½ cup	1-1.5 g
Peas	½ cup	3.5-4 g
Potato, baked	1 medium	5 g
Spinach, fresh	½ cup	1 g
Spinach, boiled	½ cup	2.5 g
Tomato, red, ripe	1 medium	1 g
Most other vegetables	½ cup	1 g

Resources: Nutritionist Pro™ Nutrition Analysis Software from Axxya Systems www.nutritionistpro.com (used with permission) and USDA Dietary Guidelines for Americans 2005 at www.health.gov/

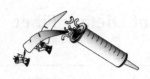

Appendix D — Food Sources of Fat

Type of Fat	Common Sources	Effect on Your Health
Monounsaturated	Extra-virgin olive oil Canola oil (120) Peanut oils, peanut butter Most nuts Avocados	Very healthful. Should be the main source of fat for most people.
Polyunsaturated	Corn oil Soybean oil Safflower oil Sunflower oil Cottonseed oil	Healthful in moderation, use sparingly.
Omega-3 fatty acids	Cold-water fish like salmon Flaxseed oil, flax seeds, flax meal Walnuts	Necessary for good health
Saturated	Whole milk Butter Cheese Cream Lard Meat fat Coconuts	These are not as healthful, but OK to use in small amounts.
Trans fats (A type of saturated fat)	Most margarines Vegetable shortening Partially hydrogenated vegetable oil	Very negative health effects. Do not use at all

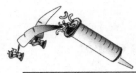

Appendix E - Food Sources of Dietary Fiber

Food, Standard Amount	Dietary Fiber (g)	Calories
Navy beans, cooked, ½ cup	9.5	128
Bran ready-to-eat cereal (100%), ½ cup	8.8	78
Kidney beans, canned, ½ cup	8.2	109
Split peas, cooked, ½ cup	8.1	116
Lentils, cooked, ½ cup	7.8	115
Black beans, cooked, ½ cup	7.5	114
Pinto beans, cooked, ½ cup	7.7	122
Lima beans, cooked, ½ cup	6.6	108
Refried beans, vegetarian, canned, ½ cup	6.5	119
Artichoke, globe, cooked, 1 each	6.5	60
White beans, canned, ½ cup	6.3	154
Chickpeas, cooked, ½ cup	6.2	135
Great northern beans, cooked, ½ cup	6.2	105
Cowpeas, cooked, ½ cup	5.6	100
Raspberries, frozen, ½ cup	5.5	129
Papaya, raw, 1 medium	5.5	119
Soybeans, mature, cooked, ½ cup	5.2	149
Bran ready-to-eat cereals, various, ~1 oz	2.6-5.0	90-108
Crackers, rye wafers, plain, 2 wafers	5.0	74
Sweet potato, baked, with skin, 1 medium (146 g)	4.8	131
Potato, baked, with skin, 1 medium	4.8	220
Asian pear, raw, 1 small	4.4	51
Green peas, cooked, ½ cup	4.4	67
Whole-wheat English muffin, 1 each	4.4	134
Pear, raw, 1 small	4.3	81
Bulgur, cooked, ½ cup	4.1	76
Mixed vegetables, cooked, ½ cup	4.0	59
Raspberries, raw, ½ cup	4.0	32
Sweet potato, boiled, no peel, 1 medium (156 g)	3.9	119
Blackberries, raw, ½ cup	3.8	31
Potato, baked, with skin, 1 medium	3.8	161
Soybeans, green, cooked, ½ cup	3.8	127
Stewed prunes, ½ cup	3.8	133
Figs, dried, ¼ cup	3.7	93

(Continued on next page.)

Appendix E—Food Sources of Dietary Fiber (Continued from previous page.)

Food, Standard Amount	Dietary Fiber (g)	Calories
Dates, ¼ cup	3.6	126
Oat bran, raw, ¼ cup	3.6	58
Pumpkin, canned, ½ cup	3.6	42
Spinach, frozen, cooked, ½ cup	3.5	30
Shredded wheat ready-to-eat cereals, ~1 oz	2.8-3.4	96
Almonds, 1 oz	3.3	164
Apple with skin, raw, 1 medium	3.3	72
Brussels sprouts, frozen, cooked, ½ cup	3.2	33
Whole-wheat spaghetti, cooked, ½ cup	3.1	87
Banana, 1 medium	3.1	105
Orange, raw, 1 medium	3.1	62
Oat bran muffin, 1 small	3.0	178
Guava, 1 medium	3.0	37
Pearled barley, cooked, ½ cup	3.0	97
Sauerkraut, canned, solids, and liquids, ½ cup	3.0	23
Raisins, seedless, ½ cup	3.0	225
Sweet potato, canned, drained, ½ cup	2.9	106
Oat bran, cooked, ½ cup	2.9	44
Tomato paste, ¼ cup	2.9	54
Winter squash, cooked, ½ cup	2.9	38
Broccoli, cooked, ½ cup	2.8	26
Parsnips, cooked, chopped, ½ cup	2.8	55
Turnip greens, cooked, ½ cup	2.5	15
Collards, cooked, ½ cup	2.7	25
Okra, frozen, cooked, ½ cup	2.6	26
Peas, edible-podded, cooked, ½ cup	2.5	42
Blueberries, frozen, ½ cup	2.4	93

Resources: Nutritionist Pro™ Nutrition Analysis Software from Axxya Systems www.nutritionistpro.com.
Used with Permission and USDA Dietary Guidelines for Americans 2005 at www.health.gov/dietaryguidelines/

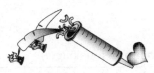

Vitamins	Common Food Sources	Promotes
Biotin	Liver, egg yolk, soybeans, milk, meat	Metabolizes amino acids and is important for hair growth
Vitamin B12 (Cyanocobalamin)	Animal foods only: meat, fish, poultry, cheese, milk, eggs, soy milk fortified with vitamin B12	Promotes building protein in the body, red blood cells and normal function of nervous tissue.
Folic acid and Folate	Yeast, liver, leafy green vegetables, oranges, cantaloupe, seeds, fortified breads and cereals (grains)	Red blood cell formation, metabolism of fats, protein synthesis
Niacin (Vitamin B3)	Milk, eggs, poultry, meat fish, whole grain, enriched cereals and grains, leafy green vegetables	Promotes energy metabolism, proper digestion and healthy nervous system
Pantothenic acid (Vitamin B5)	Meats and organ meats, fish, eggs, leafy green vegetables, legumes, whole grains, enriched food products	Promotes energy metabolism
Vitamin B6 (Pyridoxine)	Liver, meat, whole grains, legumes, potatoes	Promotes cell growth
Vitamin B2 (Riboflavin)	Meat, dairy products, eggs, green vegetables, whole grains, enriched breads and cereals	Promotes healthy skin, eyes and good energy levels
Thiamine (Vitamin B1)	Enriched cereals and breads, soybeans, lean pork, whole grains, legumes, seeds and nuts	Energy metabolism and proper functioning of the nervous system and appetite
Vitamin C (Ascorbic acid)	Papaya, citrus fruits, tomatoes, cabbage, potatoes, cantaloupe, strawberries, brcocoli, green and red peppers	Antioxidant needed for formation of collagen, promotes healthy teeth, gums and blood vessels, improves iron absorption and resistance to infection
Vitamin A	Fortified milk, liver, egg, cheese, dark green and yellow vegetables, and yellow fruits	New cell growth, healthy hair, skin and tissue and vision in dim light
Vitamin D	Fortified milk fish, liver, egg yolk, salmon	Promotes absorption and use of calcium and phosphate for healthy bones and teeth
Vitamin E	Sardines, green leafy vegetables, vegetable oils, wheat germ, whole grains, butter, liver, egg yolk	Protects red blood cells , helps prevent the destruction of vitamins A and C
Vitamin K	Cow's milk, green leafy vegetables, pork, liver, cauliflower, wheat bran	Helps blood clot properly

Modified from Pediatric Nutrition Handbook, Fifth Edition, American Academy of Pediatrics, 2004 Ronald E. Kleinman

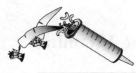

Appendix G - Food Sources of Vitamin C

Food, Standard Amount	Vitamin C (mg)	Calories
Guava, raw, ½ cup	188	56
Red sweet pepper, raw, ½ cup	142	20
Red sweet pepper, cooked, ½ cup	116	19
Kiwi fruit, 1 medium	70	46
Orange, raw, 1 medium	70	62
Orange juice, ¾ cup	61-93	79-84
Green pepper, sweet, raw, ½ cup	60	15
Green pepper, sweet, cooked, ½ cup	51	19
Grapefruit juice, ¾ cup	50-70	71-86
Vegetable juice cocktail, ¾ cup	50	34
Strawberries, raw, ½ cup	49	27
Brussels sprouts, cooked, ½ cup	48	28
Cantaloupe, ¼ medium	47	51
Papaya, raw, ¼ medium	47	30
Kohlrabi, cooked, ½ cup	45	24
Broccoli, raw, ½ cup	39	15
Edible pod peas, cooked, ½ cup	38	34
Broccoli, cooked, ½ cup	37	26
Sweet potato, canned, ½ cup	34	116
Tomato juice, ¾ cup	33	31
Tomato soup, canned, ½ cup	33	42
Cauliflower, cooked, ½ cup	28	17
Pineapple, raw, ½ cup	28	37
Kale, cooked, ½ cup	27	18
Mango, ½ cup	23	54

Resources: Nutritionist Pro™ Nutrition Analysis Software from Axxya Systems www.nutritionistpro.com
(used with permission) and USDA Dietary Guidelines for Americans 2005 at www.health.gov/dietaryguidelines/

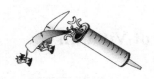

Appendix H - Food Sources of Vitamin A

Food , Standard Amount	Vitamin A (µg RAE)	Calories
Organ meats (liver, giblets), various, cooked, 3 oz	1490-9126	134-235
Carrot juice, ¾ cup	1692	71
Sweet potato with peel, baked, 1 medium	1096	103
Pumpkin, canned, ½ cup	953	42
Carrots, cooked from fresh, ½ cup	671	27
Spinach, cooked from frozen, ½ cup	573	30
Collards, cooked from frozen, ½ cup	489	31
Kale, cooked from frozen, ½ cup	478	20
Mixed vegetables, canned, ½ cup	474	40
Turnip greens, cooked from frozen, ½ cup	441	24
Instant cooked cereals, fortified, prepared, 1 packet	285-376	75-97
Various ready-to-eat cereals, with added vitamin A, ~1 oz	180-376	100-117
Carrot, raw, 1 small	301	20
Beet greens, cooked, ½ cup	276	19
Winter squash (all varieties), cooked, ½ cup	268	38
Dandelion greens, cooked, ½ cup	260	18
Cantaloupe, raw, ½ medium melon	233	46
Mustard greens, cooked, ½ cup	221	11
Pickled herring, 3 oz	219	222
Red sweet pepper, cooked, ½ cup	186	19
Chinese cabbage, cooked, ½ cup	180	10

Resources: Nutritionist Pro™ Nutrition Analysis Software from Axxya Systems www.nutritionistpro.com
(used with permission)and USDA Dietary Guidelines for Americans 2005 at www.health.gov/dietaryguidelines/

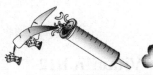

♡ Appendix I - Food Sources of Vitamin E

Food, Standard Amount	AT (mg)	Calories
Fortified ready-to-eat cereals, ~1 oz	1.6-12.8	90-107
Sunflower seeds, dry roasted, 1 oz	7.4	165
Almonds, 1 oz	7.3	164
Sunflower oil, high linoleic, 1 Tbsp	5.6	120
Cottonseed oil, 1 Tbsp	4.8	120
Safflower oil, high oleic, 1 Tbsp	4.6	120
Hazelnuts (filberts), 1 oz	4.3	178
Mixed nuts, dry roasted, 1 oz	3.1	168
Turnip greens, frozen, cooked, ½ cup	2.9	24
Tomato paste, ¼ cup	2.8	54
Pine nuts, 1 oz	2.6	191
Peanut butter, 2 Tbsp	2.5	192
Tomato puree, ½ cup	2.5	48
Tomato sauce, ½ cup	2.5	39
Canola oil, 1 Tbsp	2.4	124
Wheat germ, toasted, plain, 2 Tbsp	2.3	54
Mango, raw, 1 whole	2.3	135
Peanuts, 1 oz	2.2	166
Avocado, raw, ½ medium	2.1	161
Carrot juice, canned, ¾ cup	2.1	71
Peanut oil, 1 Tbsp	2.1	119
Corn oil, 1 Tbsp	1.9	120
Olive oil, 1 Tbsp	1.9	119
Spinach, cooked, ½ cup	1.9	21
Dandelion greens, cooked, ½ cup	1.8	18
Sardine, Atlantic, in oil, drained, 3 oz	1.7	177
Blue crab, cooked/canned, 3 oz	1.6	84
Brazil nuts, 1 oz	1.6	186
Herring, Atlantic, pickled, 3 oz	1.5	222
Apricots, canned, drained, with skin, 1 cup	1.5	150
Margarine, regular, 1 Tbsp	1.3	100
Broccoli, frozen, chopped, cooked ½ cup	1.2	25
Peaches, canned or raw, 1 cup	1.2	74

Resources: Nutritionist Pro™ Nutrition Analysis Software from Axxya Systems www.nutritionistpro.com
(used with permission)and USDA Dietary Guidelines for Americans 2005 at www.health.gov/dietaryguidelines/

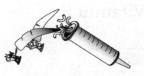

Appendix J - Food Sources of Vitamin B12

Food, Standard Amount	Vitamin B12 Micrograms (µg) per serving	Percent Daily Value
Liver, beef, braised, 1 slice	47.9	780
Fortified breakfast cereals (100% fortified), ¾ cup	6.0	100
Trout, rainbow, wild, cooked, 3 oz	5.4	90
Salmon, sockeye, cooked, 3 oz	4.9	80
Trout, rainbow, farmed, cooked, 3 oz	4.2	50
Beef, top sirloin, lean, choice, broiled, 3 oz	2.4	40
Fortified breakfast cereals (25% fortified), ¾ cup	1.5	25
Yogurt, plain, skim, with 13 grams protein per cup, 1 cup	1.4	25
Haddock, cooked, 3 oz	1.2	20
Clams, breaded & fried, ¾ cup	1.1	20
Tuna, white, canned in water, drained, solids, 3 oz	1.0	15
Milk, 1 cup	0.9	15
Pork, cured, ham, lean only, canned, roasted, 3 oz	0.6	10
Egg, whole, hard boiled, 1	0.6	10
American pasteurized cheese food, 1 oz	0.3	6
Chicken, breast, meat only, roasted, ½ breast	0.3	6

Resources: Nutritionist Pro™ Nutrition Analysis Software from Axxya Systems www.nutritionistpro.com (used with permission) and USDA Dietary Guidelines for Americans 2005 at www.health.gov/dietaryguidelines/

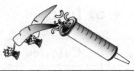

Appendix K - Mineral Chart

Mineral	Common Food Sources	Promotes
Calcium	Milk and milk products, broccoli, cabbage, kale, tofu, sardines and salmon	Healthy bones and teeth, normal blood clotting and nervous system function
Chromium	Corn oil, clams, whole grain cereals, brewer's yeast	Energy (glucose metabolism), increases effectiveness of insulin
Copper	Oysters, shellfish, nuts, organ meats, legumes, green leafy vegetables	Synthesis of hemoglobin, proper iron metabolism and maintenance of blood vessels
Iodine	Seafood, iodized salt	Component of thyroxin central to metabolism
Iron	Meats and organ meats, fish, eggs, leafy green vegetables, legumes, whole grains, enriched food products	Hemoglobin formation, improves blood quality, increases resistance to stress and disease.
Magnesium	Nuts, green vegetables, whole grains, dairy products, meat, fish, poultry, legumes	Healthy bones and teeth, proper nervous system functioning and energy metabolism
Manganese	Whole grains, vegetables, fruits, tea	Enzyme structure
Phosphorous	Fish, lean meat, poultry, eggs, grains, milk	Healthy bones and teeth, energy metabolism, acid /base balance
Potassium	Bananas, raisins, apricots, oranges, avocados, dates, melons, prunes, broccoli, spinach, carrots, potatoes, winter squash, mushrooms, peas, lentils, dried beans, peanuts, milk, yogurt, lean meats	Fluid balance, activity of heart muscle, nervous system and kidneys
Selenium	Seafood, organ meats, grains	Protects body tissue against oxidative damage from radiation, pollutions and normal metabolic processing
Zinc	Lean meats, seafood, liver, eggs, milk, legumes, whole grains	Promotes cell reproduction, tissue growth and repair

Adapted from the American Institute for Cancer Research

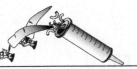

Appendix L - Food Sources of Iron

Food, Standard Amount	Iron (mg)	Calories
Clams, canned, drained, 3 oz	23.8	126
Fortified ready-to-eat cereals (various), ~ 1 oz	1.8 -21.1	54-127
Oysters, Eastern, wild, cooked with moist heat, 3 oz	10.2	116
Organ meats (liver, giblets), various, cooked, 3 oz	5.2-9.9	134-235
Fortified, instant, cooked cereals (various), 1 packet	4.9-8.1	Varies
Soybeans, mature, cooked, ½ cup	4.4	149
Pumpkin and squash seed kernels, roasted, 1 oz	4.2	148
White beans, canned, ½ cup	3.9	153
Blackstrap molasses, 1 Tbsp	3.5	47
Lentils, cooked, ½ cup	3.3	115
Spinach, cooked from fresh, ½ cup	3.2	21
Beef, chuck, blade roast, lean, cooked, 3 oz	3.1	215
Beef, bottom round, lean, 0" fat, all grades, cooked, 3 oz	2.8	182
Kidney beans, cooked, ½ cup	2.6	112
Sardines, canned in oil, drained, 3 oz	2.5	177
Oat bran, raw, ½ cup	2.5	116
Beef, rib, lean, ¼" fat, all grades, 3 oz	2.4	195
Chickpeas, cooked, ½ cup	2.4	134
Duck, meat only, roasted, 3 oz	2.3	171
Lamb, shoulder, arm, lean, ¼" fat, choice, cooked, 3 oz	2.3	237
Prune juice, ¾ cup	2.3	136
Shrimp, canned, 3 oz	2.3	102
Cowpeas, cooked, ½ cup	2.2	100
Ground beef, 15% fat, cooked, 3 oz	2.2	212
Tomato puree, ½ cup	2.2	48
Lima beans, cooked, ½ cup	2.2	108
Soybeans, green, cooked, ½ cup	2.2	127
Navy beans, cooked, ½ cup	2.1	127
Refried beans, ½ cup	2.1	118
Beef, top sirloin, lean, 0" fat, all grades, cooked, 3 oz	2.0	156
Tomato paste, ¼ cup	2.0	54

Resource: USDA Dietary Guidelines for Americans 2005 at www.health.gov/dietaryguidelines/

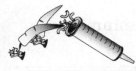

Appendix M - Food Sources of Magnesium

Food, Standard Amount	Magnesium (mg)	Calories
Pumpkin and squash seed kernels, roasted, 1 oz	151	148
Brazil nuts, 1 oz	107	186
Bran ready-to-eat cereal (100%), ~1 oz	103	74
Halibut, cooked, 3 oz	91	119
Quinoa, dry, ¼ cup	89	159
Spinach, canned, ½ cup	81	25
Almonds, 1 oz	78	164
Spinach, cooked from fresh, ½ cup	78	20
Buckwheat flour, ¼ cup	75	101
Cashews, dry roasted, 1 oz	74	163
Soybeans, mature, cooked, ½ cup	74	149
Pine nuts, dried, 1 oz	71	191
Mixed nuts, oil roasted, with peanuts, 1 oz	67	175
White beans, canned, ½ cup	67	154
Pollock, walleye, cooked, 3 oz	62	96
Black beans, cooked, ½ cup	60	114
Bulgur, dry, ¼ cup	57	120
Oat bran, raw, ¼ cup	55	58
Soybeans, green, cooked, ½ cup	54	127
Tuna, yellowfin, cooked, 3 oz	54	118
Artichokes (hearts), cooked, ½ cup	50	42
Peanuts, dry roasted, 1 oz	50	166
Lima beans, baby, cooked from frozen, ½ cup	50	95
Beet greens, cooked, ½ cup	49	19
Navy beans, cooked, ½ cup	48	127
Tofu, firm, prepared with nigari*, ½ cup	47	88
Okra, cooked from frozen, ½ cup	47	26
Soy beverage, 1 cup	47	127
Cowpeas, cooked, ½ cup	46	100
Hazelnuts, 1 oz	46	178
Oat bran muffin, 1 oz	45	77
Great northern beans, cooked, ½ cup	44	104
Oat bran, cooked, ½ cup	44	44
Buckwheat groats, roasted, cooked, ½ cup	43	78
Brown rice, cooked, ½ cup	42	108
Haddock, cooked, 3 oz	42	95

* Calcium sulfate and magnesium chloride
Resource: USDA Dietary Guidelines for Americans 2005 at www.health.gov/dietaryguidelines/

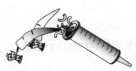

Appendix N - Sources of Potassium

Food, Standard Amount	Potassium (mg)	Calories
Sweet potato, baked, 1 potato (146 g)	694	131
Tomato paste, ¼ cup	664	54
Beet greens, cooked, ½ cup	655	19
Potato, baked, flesh, 1 potato (156 g)	610	145
White beans, canned, ½ cup	595	153
Yogurt, plain, non-fat, 8-oz container	579	127
Raisins, seedless, ½ cup	563	225
Tomato puree, ½ cup	549	48
Dates, Deglet Noor, 10 whole dates	541	228
Clams, canned, 3 oz	534	126
Yogurt, plain, low-fat, 8-oz container	531	143
Artichokes, cooked, boiled, drained, ½ medium	531	75
Prune juice, ¾ cup	530	136
Carrot juice, ¾ cup	517	71
Blackstrap molasses, 1 Tbsp	498	47
Halibut, cooked, 3 oz	490	119
Soybeans, green, cooked, ½ cup	485	127
Tuna, yellowfin, cooked, 3 oz	484	118
Lima beans, cooked, ½ cup	484	104
Squash, (winter & all varieties), cooked, ½ cup	448	40
Rockfish, Pacific, cooked, 3 oz	442	103
Cod, Pacific, cooked, 3 oz	439	89
Evaporated milk, nonfat, canned, ½ cup	425	100
Bananas, 1 medium	422	105
Spinach, cooked, ½ cup	419	21
Tomato juice, ¾ cup	417	31
Tomato sauce, ½ cup	405	39

(Continued on next page.)

Appendix N—Sources of Potassium (Continued from previous page.)

Food, Standard Amount	Potassium (mg)	Calories
Peaches, dried, uncooked, ¼ cup	398	96
Prunes, stewed, ½ cup	398	133
Papaya, ½ medium	391	60
Milk, non-fat, 1 cup	382	83
Pork chop, center loin, cooked, 3 oz	382	197
Apricots, dried, uncooked, ¼ cup	378	78
Navy beans, cooked, ½ cup	378	148
Rainbow trout, farmed, cooked, 3 oz	375	144
Pork loin, center rib (roasts), lean, roasted, 3 oz	371	190
Buttermilk, cultured, low-fat, 1 cup	370	98
Cantaloupe, ¼ medium	368	47
Milk, 1%-2%, 1 cup	366	102-122
Honeydew melon, ⅛ medium	365	58
Lentils, cooked, ½ cup	365	115
Plantains, cooked, ½ cup slices	358	90
Kidney beans, cooked, ½ cup	358	112
Orange juice, ¾ cup	355	85
Split peas, cooked, ½ cup	355	116
Yogurt, plain, whole milk, 8 oz container	352	138

Resources: Nutritionist Pro™ Nutrition Analysis Software from Axxya Systems www.nutritionistpro.com
(used with permission) and USDA Dietary Guidelines for Americans 2005 at www.health.gov/dietaryguidelines/

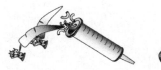

Appendix O - Food Sources Of Calcium

Food, Standard Amount	Calcium (mg)	Calories
Fortified ready-to-eat cereals (various), 1 oz	236-1043	88-106
Plain yogurt, non-fat (13 g protein/8 oz), 8-oz container	452	127
Romano cheese, 1.5 oz	452	165
Pasteurized processed Swiss cheese, 2 oz	438	190
Plain yogurt, low-fat (12 g protein/8 oz), 8-oz container	415	143
Soy beverage, calcium fortified, 1 cup	368	98
Evaporated milk, nonfat, ½ cup	371	100
Fruit yogurt, low-fat (10 g protein/8 oz), 8-oz container	345	232
Swiss cheese, 1.5 oz	336	162
Ricotta cheese, part skim, ½ cup	335	170
Eggnog, 1 cup	330	342
Sardines, Atlantic, in oil, drained, 3 oz	325	177
Pasteurized processed American cheese food, 2 oz	323	188
Provolone cheese, 1.5 oz	321	150
Mozzarella cheese, part-skim, 1.5 oz	311	129
Cheddar cheese, 1.5 oz	307	171
Fat-free (skim) milk, 1 cup	306	83
Muenster cheese, 1.5 oz	305	156
Milk, low fat (1%), 1 cup	290	102
Milk, chocolate, low fat (1%), 1 cup	288	158
Milk, reduced fat (2%), 1 cup	285	122
Milk, chocolate, reduced fat (2%), 1 cup	285	180
Milk, buttermilk, low fat (1%), 1 cup	284	98
Milk, whole, 1 cup	276	146
Milk, chocolate, whole, 1 cup	280	208
Yogurt, plain, whole milk (8 g protein/8 oz), 8-oz container	275	138
Ricotta cheese, whole milk, ½ cup	255	214
Tofu, firm, prepared with nigari* , ½ cup	253	88
Blue cheese, 1.5 oz	225	150
Mozzarella cheese, whole milk, 1.5 oz	215	128
Feta cheese, 1.5 oz	210	113
Pink salmon, canned, with bone, 3 oz	181	118

194   (Continued on next page.)

Appendix O—Food Sources of Calcium (Continued from previous page.)

Food, Standard Amount	Calcium (mg)	Calories
Collards, cooked from frozen, ½ cup	178	31
Rhubarb, cooked from frozen, ½ cup	174	139
Molasses, blackstrap, 1 Tbsp	172	47
Spinach, cooked from frozen, ½ cup	146	30
Soybeans, green, cooked, ½ cup	130	127
Turnip greens, cooked from frozen, ½ cup	124	24
Ocean perch, Atlantic, cooked, 3 oz	116	103
Oatmeal, plain and flavored, instant, fortified, 1 packet prepared	99-110	97-157
Cowpeas, cooked, ½ cup	106	80
White beans, canned, ½ cup	96	153
Kale, cooked from frozen, ½ cup	90	20
Okra, cooked from frozen, ½ cup	88	26
Soybeans, mature, cooked, ½ cup	88	149
Blue crab, canned, 3 oz	86	84
Beet greens, cooked from fresh, ½ cup	82	19
Bok Choy, Chinese cabbage, cooked from fresh, ½ cup	79	10
Clams, canned, 3 oz	78	126
Cottage cheese, lowfat, ½ cup	78	102
Dandelion greens, cooked from fresh, ½ cup	74	17
Rainbow trout, farmed, cooked, 3 oz	73	144

* Calcium sulfate and magnesium chloride.

Resources: Nutritionist Pro™ Nutrition Analysis Software from Axxya Systems www.nutritionistpro.com
(used with permission)and USDA Dietary Guidelines for Americans 2005 at www.health.gov/dietaryguidelines/

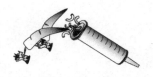

Appendix P - Food Sources of Milk and Milk Substitutes

Milk/ Milk Substitutes	Amount	Calories	Protein	Fat	Carbo	Calcium
Whole milk	1 cup	150	8 g	8 g	11 g	276 mg
Skim milk	1 cup	85	8 g	0 g	12 g	302 mg
2% milk	1 cup	120	8 g	5 g	11 g	285 mg
1% milk	1 cup	100	8 g	3 g	11 g	290 mg
Evaporated whole milk	1 cup	300-400	17-18 g	10 g	13 g	329 mg
Soy milk	1 cup	80-120	7 g	3 g	8 g	368 mg
Rice milk	1 cup	120	1 g	3 g	22 g	300 mg
Goat milk	1 cup	168	9 g	10 g	11 g	326 mg
Almond milk	1 cup	70	2 g	3 g	1 g	240 mg
Coconut milk, canned	1 cup	445	5 g	48 g	6 g	41 mg
Nonfat dry milk, prepared	1 cup	81	8 g	0 g	11.8 g	279 mg
Nonfat dry milk, powder	1 Tbsp	16-27	1.5-2.5 g	0 g	2-4 g	53-95 mg
Yogurt, plain from whole milk	1 cup	140-180	7-13 g	7.4g	11 g	300 mg

Resources: Nutritionist Pro™ Nutrition Analysis Software from Axxya Systems www.nutritionistpro.com
(used with permission) and USDA Dietary Guidelines for Americans 2005 at www.health.gov/dietaryguidelines/

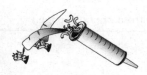

Food Component	Common Sources
Milk Protein (Casein)	Milk (including cow milk, goat milk, powdered milk, condensed, buttermilk and canned milk) Milk solids, milk protein, milk derivatives, malted milk, and dried milk solids Butter, butter fat, butter-flavored oil, butter solids, ghee, artificial butter flavor, natural butter flavor Cheese – hard, soft, creamed and processed Sour cream, sour cream solids Cream, whipped cream, half-and-half, light cream Cottage cheese, yogurt, ice cream, ice milk, sherbet Whey, whey powder, whey protein, whey protein hydrolysate, hydrolysed whey, delactosed whey, demineralized whey, milk protein hydrolysate, sweet dairy whey Lactose, lactalbumin, lactoglobulin, lactulose, lactalbumin phosphate Caseinates, casein, casei, casein hydrolysate, hydroloysed casein, ammonium caseinate, calcium caseinate, potassium caseinate, sodium caseinate, and rennet casein Calcium lactate (verify from the manufacturer that it is not derived from dairy) Nisin (used in countries other than the U.S. and contains casein)
Gluten	Wheat products: Wheat, wheat berries, wheat bran, wheat grass, wheat germ, wheat nut, wheat starch, wheaten, bulgar, couscous, dinkle durum, dinkom, emmer, fanna®, faro, FU, graham flour, kamut, matza, matzo, matzoh, MIR, orzo, seitan, semolina, spelt and triticale. Oat Products: Oat, oat bran, oat fiber, oat gum, oat syrup Barley products: Barley, malt, malt extract, malt flavoring, malt liquor, malt syrup, malt vinegar Gluten products: Gluten, rye, filler, gliadin
Corn (continued next page)	If a child is highly allergic to corn, it is safest to avoid the oil derived from it. Corn oil may become contaminated with corn protein during manufacturing. The following foods either contain corn, or have the possibility of containing a corn product. Read labels carefully. Artificial flavoring Ascorbic acid (vitamin C), Aspartame (Nutrasweet®) Caramel coloring Corn products including corn: corn alcohol, corn extract, corn syrup, corn syrup solids Corn, cane or beet sugar Carob Citric acid Dextrin (corn, wheat or tapioca) Dextrates or dextrose Food starch Glycerines (corn oil) Fructose (corn or fruit) Generic alcohol Gluten (corn or wheat or animal fat) Golden syrup (treacle, corn or molasses) High fructose corn syrup Hydrolyzed corn or vegetable protein Iodized table salt

Food Component	Common Sources
Corn (Continued from previous page)	Invert sugars or invert syrups Lactic acid lecithin (corn or soy) Malt (corn or barley) Maltodextrin Maple flavoring (corn, gluten or soy) Modified food starch MSG Natural flavoring (root beer, corn or gluten) Nut flavoring Saccharin Sorbitol ® Starch Treacle Textured vegetable protein Vegetable oil vinegar Xanthan gum
Soy Protein	Most of these foods and food components contain soy protein. *Read the label.* Akara Edamame Hydrolyzed vegetable protein Hydrolyzed protein Kyodufu (freeze dried tofu) Luncheon meats Miso Natto Okara (soy pulp) Pork link sausages Salad dressings (Some) Sauces Shoyu Sobee Soy products including albumin, soy, soybean, soy bran, soy beverages, soy butter, soy cheese, soy flour, soy grits, soybean paste, soy meal, soy milk soy, nuts, soy oil, soy pasta, soy protein, soy protein concentrate, soy protein isolate, soy sauce, soy sprouts Supro Taman Tempeh Teriaki Textured vegetable protein Tofu Vegan cheese Vegetable oil (Some) vitamins, vitamin E Yuba

Share Your Thoughts

This book has been a compilation of ideas and experiences from parents and professionals who understand how to tube feed children. The body of knowledge and research in this area is evolving. If you have a thought to share, your experience, a recipe, or a technique which will make tube feeding easier for another family, or if you have information you would like another parent or professional to know, PLEASE take a moment to fill out and return this comment page. We will consider these ideas when the book is revised in the future.

Comments:

_____

_____

_____

_____

_____

_____

_____

_____

_____

_____

_____

_____

_____

_____

_____

_____

_____

Name _____

Email _____

Address _____

Phone _____

(Your name and address are optional. It helps us contact you if we have questions.)

Return to: Feedback, Mealtime Notions, LLC . PO 35432, Tucson, AZ 85740

Homemade Blended Formula Handbook

Homemade Blended Formula Handbook offers the reader an integral way of thinking about providing meals for tube fed children—meals that are nourishing physically, mentally, and emotionally. At its deepest level this is a book about children and their families. It is a book about mealtimes as a focal point in the life of the child, family and community.

The primary focus is to offer a deep understanding of how to create tube feeding meals that are compiled from foods that are available to all children and families. It provides a guide to the process from the initial concept to the development of formulas that offer dietary diversity and high-level nutrition. It looks at homemade blended formula options on a continuum which identifies the best fit for each child and each family.

It offers practical ways of including children who receive their nutrition by feeding tube into the life of the mealtime community. It celebrates their unique contributions, in partnership with the person who feeds them.

Homemade Blended Formula Handbook is for families and professionals who together are making the choice to try homemade blended formulas for tube feeding.

Mealtime Notions, LLC
P.O. Box 35432
Tucson, AZ 85740
www.mealtimenotions.com

Made in the USA
Las Vegas, NV
17 February 2024